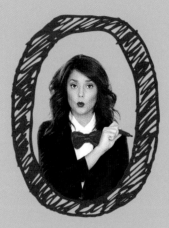

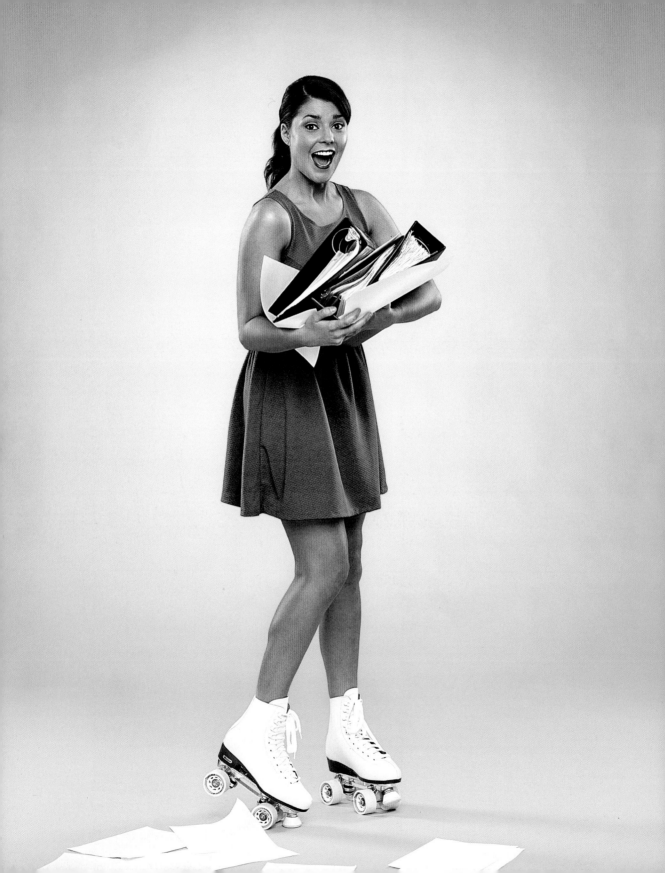

GRACE'S GUIDE

THE ART OF PRETENDING TO BE A GROWN-UP

By
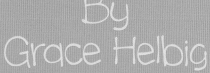
Grace Helbig

A Touchstone Book

Published by Simon & Schuster

New York   London   Toronto   Sydney   New Delhi

Touchstone

A Division of Simon & Schuster, Inc.
1230 Avenue of the Americas
New York, NY 10020

Interior design by Shawn Dahl, dahlimama inc
Illustrations by Alison Oliver, Sugar
Photos by Robin Roemer

First Touchstone trade paperback edition October 2014

TOUCHSTONE and colophon are registered trademarks of
Simon & Schuster, Inc.

For information about special discounts for bulk purchases,
please contact Simon & Schuster Special Sales at
1-866-506-1949 or business@simonandschuster.com.

The Simon & Schuster Speakers Bureau can bring
authors to your live event. For more information or to
book an event, contact the Simon & Schuster Speakers
Bureau at 1-866-248-3049 or visit our website at
www.simonspeakers.com.

Manufactured in the United States of America

10 9 8 7 6 5 4 3

Library of Congress Cataloging-in-Publication Data
Helbig, Grace.
   Grace's guide : the art of pretending to be a grown-up /
Grace Helbig.
      pages cm
1. Young adults—Humor. 2. Adulthood—Humor.
3. Conduct of life—Humor. I. Title.
   PN6231.A26H45 2014
   818'.602—dc23
                              2014023166
ISBN 978-1-4767-8800-5
ISBN 978-1-4767-8802-9 (ebook)

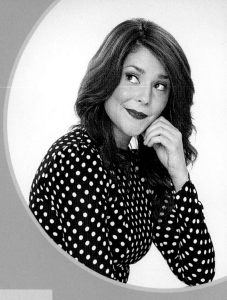

For the anxious, awkward, wonderful weirds
who constantly inspire me.

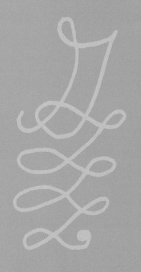

CONTENTS

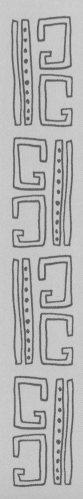

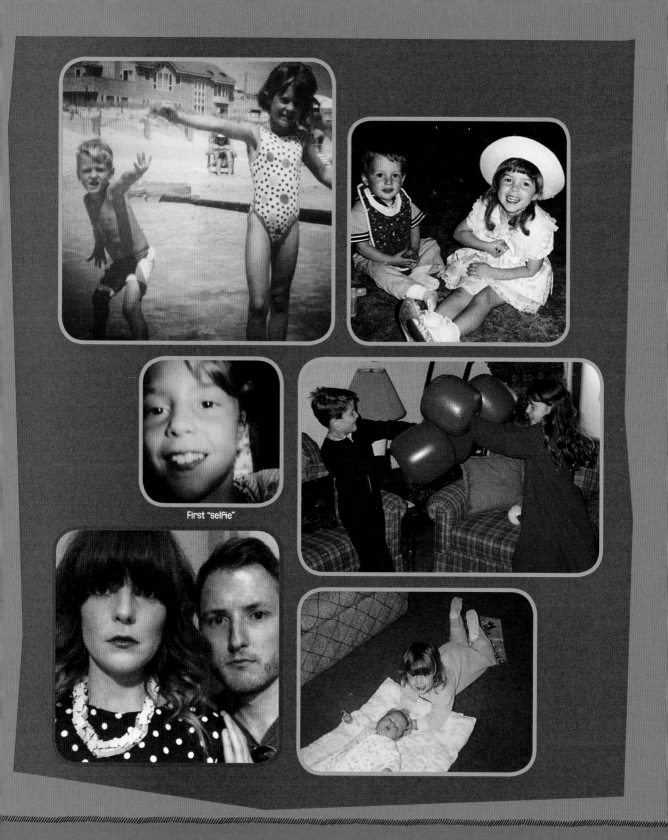

First "selfie"

FOREWORD

Ali/Frazier. Red Sox/Yankees. Navratilova/Evert. Babe Ruth/mild physical activity. Many consider these to be some of the greatest sports rivalries in history. But are they?

The only legendary rivalry that interests me is the one between Tim Helbig (me) and Grace Helbig in the sport of kings: Nintendo 64's sushi-go-round mini-game in Pokémon Stadium.

For those of you who don't know, sushi-go-round is a game where you play a Lickitung (Pokémon #108) racing to outspend your opponents by "eating" sushi of various prices that are circling on a conveyor belt around your Pokémon. The fact that I even have to explain what sushi-go-round is reveals the abhorrent state of our educational system. (What are they even teaching you in school these days?)

Grace, my older sister of two years, and I were fervent sushi-go-round players, and not a weekend went by in the early to mid-2000s when we weren't poised with our N64 controllers, sitting uncomfortably next to a pool table our parents thought we wanted for some reason. The rivalry was heated, and we were prone to sabotage. She would push me into eating a sushi roll that would break my combo; I would nudge her into swallowing a vat of wasabi, causing her Lickitung to convulse wildly.

We seemed to be constantly competing as kids, whether in soccer or ultimate Frisbee or for our parents' love, and this resulted in a lot of tears (almost all of them mine). Grace has always been a ruthless competitor. I remember, one time, she kicked sand in my eyes so that she would win a race on the beach. She really didn't even have to, either—those were what could best be described as "My Chubby Years" and, unless the race was consuming a bag of sandy Doritos, I was no real threat.

But we weren't always rivals; sometimes we were on the same team. When we were little, Grace and I used to play basketball against our dad. Grace devised a play called The Screaming Banshee, wherein we would scream from the back of the court and hand off the ball to each other while zigzagging toward the basket. It failed as a play, because apparently in basketball you have to dribble, but I've never screamed or laughed so hard in my life.

I'd like to think this mix of competition and teamwork with Grace turned me into the person I am today. And now Grace has written a book to help do for you what she did for me. And why shouldn't she have written it? She's got ALL THE CREDENTIALS.

Just like the Screaming Banshee play, *Grace's Guide* is her unique—and sometimes questionable—take on the game of life. Whether you're winning or losing, Grace will keep you laughing. She always has for me.

—Tim Helbig
May 2014

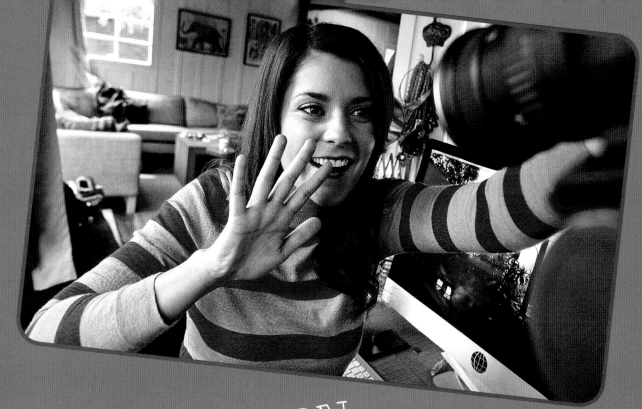

INTRODUCTION

Hello, beautiful stranger. **My name is Grace Helbig,** otherwise known as it'sGrace on that smorgasbord of digital tubes frequently referred to as the Internet.

I have a comedic vlog (video + blog = vlog . . . inform your parents) on YouTube. It's been happening for about six years now and in that time I've amassed a library (ew, what's a library? Jk. GO BOOKS!) of over a thousand videos ranging on topics from how to make nachos with mac and cheese to critiquing Barack Obama's fashion choices to teaching my viewers how to fall down in public.

I sometimes consider myself to be the Internet's awkward older sister. **I may not have ALL the answers,** but I've got my own advice, opinions, and theories to help get you through this arbitrary piss den called life.

I'm the only girl in a family of four brothers and I'm the product of a very emotionally repressed British family. Growing up, I was incredibly insecure about expressing my feelings and interacting socially.

As soon as my family got the Internet installed when I was in seventh grade, I finally found my personal paradise. I could ask questions I was too afraid to ask, research problems I was too embarrassed to bring up to my parents, and interact with individuals I'd normally be too insecure to engage with.

It became my nonjudgmental parent away from my parents. But the Internet wasn't always the best guide. I would search for advice or answers and quickly stumble into some racy, weird, highly inappropriate, disturbing, and/or nonapplicable yet fascinating information. I learned what (anal) sex was. I learned that there were entire chat rooms dedicated to suicide. I learned you could embed a code on your GeoCities website that made glitter shoot out of the mouse pointer. I learned you could learn a lot about people you barely knew.

Even though I had the entire world at my fingertips, for most of my girlhood I felt very alone. If I had had a guidebook like this one back then, maybe things might have been different (cough cough, sorry, the air is very dry in here).

I've led a relatively normal, anxiety-ridden life and I'm excited to share all of the ups and downs (reminds me I want to buy myself a trampoline) that have shaped me into the person I've become over the years; the person that sometimes finagles a grocery bag into a shirt as a means to teach girls how to do the walk of shame without shame.

I'm here to support you. I'm here to help you grow and to remind you that stupid is fun and failure is rewarding. Listen, I won't tell your mom you puked in her Jetta last Thursday. This is a self-help book that went to happy hour.

What you're about to read is (hopefully) a fun and funny Millennial's handbook. It's everything you need to know, from surviving a breakup to surviving a hangover (shockingly, those two have very similar healing methods).

Grace's Guide can be read start to finish or you can flip around—it's reader's choice! At the end of many of the chapters you'll see an acronym (like DANCE CROTCH) to help you remember the tips I just discussed. Sprinkled throughout the book you'll also find little words of wisdom from my mom (truly from my mom) and fun "Grace Notes" worksheets you can fill out. Share your "Grace Notes" with me online!

I'm going to try to help you with school, work, social activities, and lifestyle stuff to the best of my dubious abilities. Trust me, I don't have definitive answers, but I do have plenty of misadventures and lessons learned the hard way to share. Let us begin.

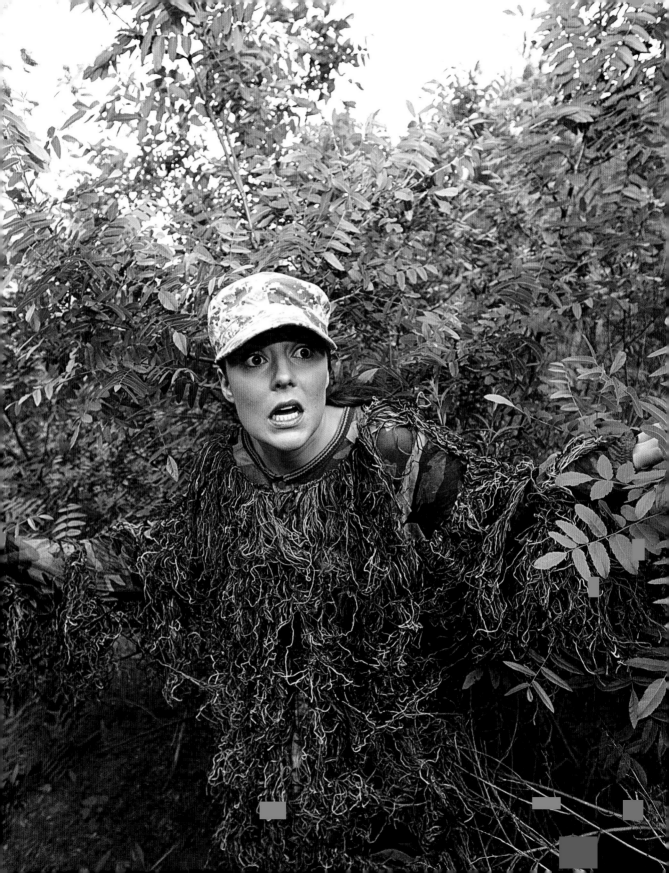

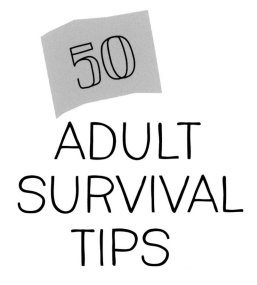

ADULT SURVIVAL TIPS

Being an adult is both super cool and super scary. You can eat ice cream whenever you want, but you might also develop a lactose issue. You can drive a car across the country if you feel like it, but you'll probably have to pay for your own car insurance. It's amazing and awful!

But there's no need to be discouraged, you skin-covered meat puppet of potential. I'm here to help. Sort of. Take all of this advice with a grain of salt. But watch your sodium levels. I'm no expert. Definitely not in life. But who is? I'm trying to get through it just like you. So what you're about to read are some of my thoughts, theories, and reflections on living a life that isn't entirely terrible. Think of this as the CliffsNotes version of my book.

Here are my fifty overall adult survival tips:

1. **Deodorant CAN be perfume.** This was almost the title of the book. I carry travel-sized deodorants in my bags, because I'm self-conscious about how I smell and I'm forgetful when it comes to basic hygiene.

2. **Never trust a middle-aged man named "Josh."** Unless he's your Russian body-guard at a YouTube convention. True story. The most stereotypical sixtyish-year-old Russian-looking man I'd ever seen, in a sleek suit and expensive glasses, walked over and introduced himself to me as my bodyguard for the meet-and-greet event I was doing. I immediately

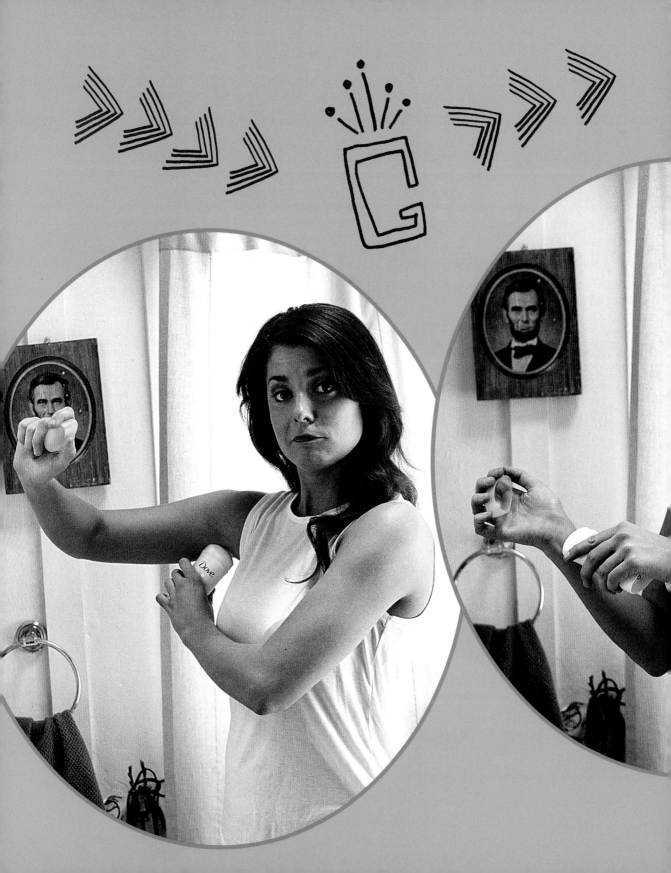

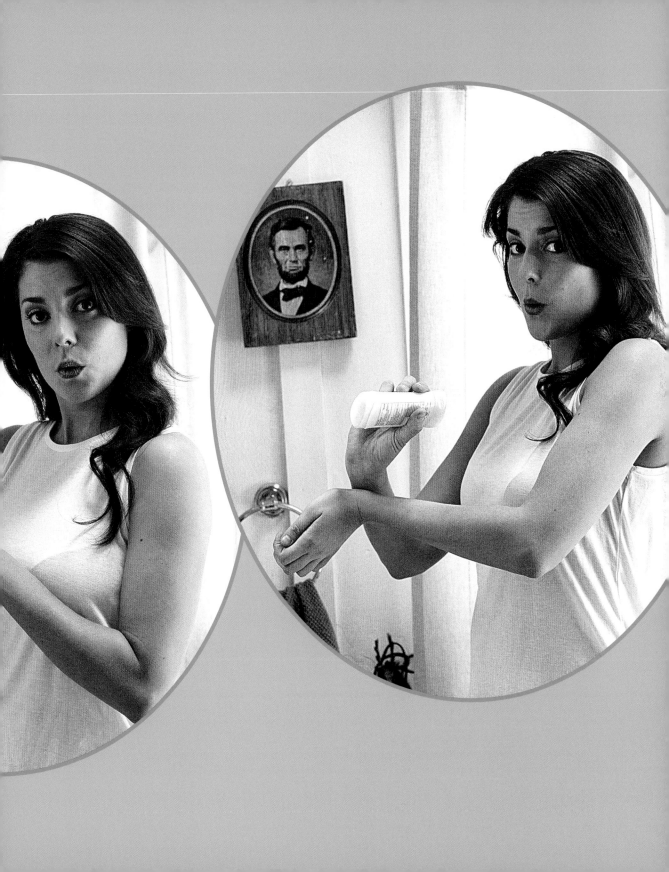

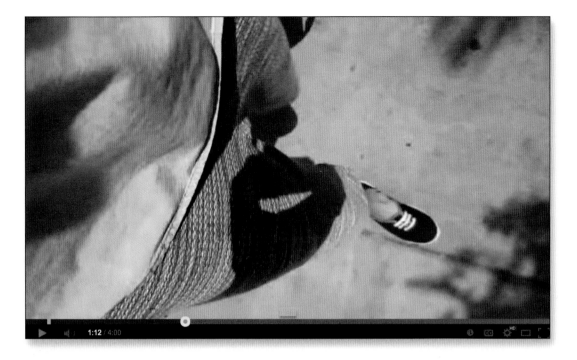

`1:12 / 4:00`

thought to myself, *This guy has killed a man*. He had that too-calm, calm vibe like he could just touch a pressure point on my shoulder and knock me out. I said, "Hi, I'm Grace," and he replied, "I'm Josh." Um, excuse me, what? Josh? This Russian man with a full Russian accent and just-shined shoes and an expensive ring that I figured was an association with his Mafia ties because I take stereotypes too far was named JOSH? Josh is supposed to be the name of a slightly attractive yet still pretty generic teenage Abercrombie & Fitch model. Long story short, Josh was great and loved whiskey. But I still don't trust middle-aged men named Josh.

3. **Wear socks.** If your shoes are supposed to be worn with socks, WEAR SOCKS. I should take my own advice. My feet staaaank. And yes, I have put deodorant on my feet before attending social events.

4. **Do your taxes.** Just do them. And don't be afraid to ask someone for help. They are confusing and annoying and UGH. But just get them done.

5. **Have spare keys.** Either hidden somewhere near your place of shelter or with your introverted friend that you can always trust to be home. Also it's helpful to have a backup plan to get into your place if somehow the keys are gone or your hermit friend got a wild haircut and went out. Can you go through a window? Pick the lock? Be prepared; you never know when your digestive tract is going to turn on you and you'll need to get into your place ASAP (oops).

6. **Make sure you have your wallet and phone.** Before you get out of a cab just take

three extra seconds to check. I've left my phone in many a cab, and it sucks. And then your needy friend is all like, *Why isn't she texting me back, did I do something wrong, she hates me, well now I hate her, this friendship is over forever, I will never forget this, I'm emotionally scarred for life.* Take a little extra time.

7. There's a YouTube video tutorial for that. You can find a YouTube tutorial for ANY-THING. I learned how to open a bottle of wine with a shoe! Yes, it took me over an hour and, yes, I later realized I could have purchased a bottle opener from the convenience store down the street, but it worked and I felt smart and resourceful and powerful.

8. Tell the cop there was a spider in your car. It's worth at least trying to explain to a cop that you were driving fast/crazy because of a really big spider. Or a bee. Or a wasp. Or you had to sneeze. Or you have explosive diarrhea. Or your vagina is bleeding. Get creative!

9. Just drink at least one goddamn glass of water a day. And then pat yourself on the back for doing something your parents can be proud of.

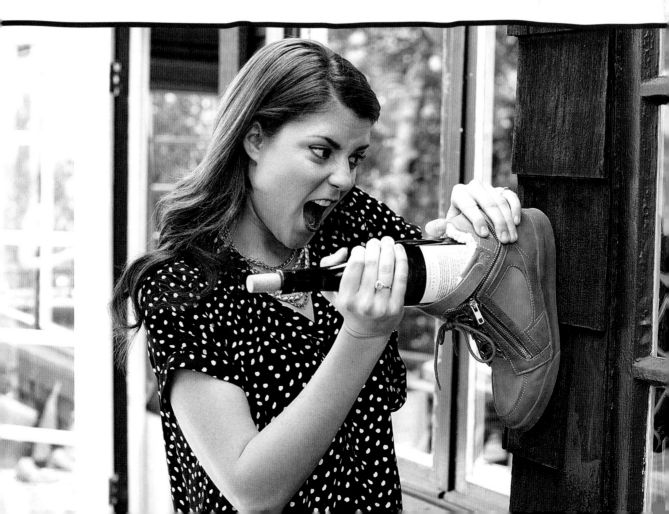

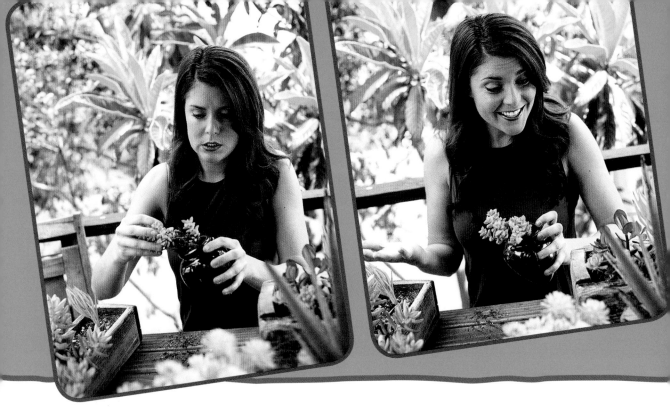

10. **Invest in a box of thank-you cards.** Old people really, really want thank-you cards. I learned that the hard way. Eeeeesh.

11. **You can get it at Target.**

12. **You probably don't want that tattoo with the flames behind it.** Imagine seeing an old man or woman in an elderly home with that tattoo. Would you be like, *Whoa, I bet there's a super-cool story behind that*, or would you be like, *Whoa, I bet they were really desperate to be cool and interesting when they were younger?*

13. **Don't be friends with someone who still "pokes" people on Facebook.** They're either your aunt or a serial killer trying to imitate normal human interaction.

14. **That really complicated Starbucks order doesn't make you interesting.** It makes you annoying. Coffee is coffee. It wakes up your brain and your butt. Just get a milkshake.

15. **Invest in at least two decent pairs of jeans/pants and two pairs of sweatpants.** It's apparently "inappropriate" to wear sweatpants to business meetings. But if you ever come to a business meeting at my place, it'll be inappropriate not to.

16. **Plants can trick people into thinking you have your sh*t together.** A little bit of greenery in your home/office says, "Oh, I'm sophisticated. I'm the kind of person that likes nature and ambience and can maintain a living plant." I'd suggest starting with something like a cactus that needs zero maintenance.

17. Build credit/get a credit card/pay off your credit card. I'm still working on this. I can't even finish making a to-do list, let alone remember to pay off a credit card. But apparently it's an important life thing. Apparently you have to have "credit" to get "approved" for "loans" to buy things like "houses" and "cars" and other things you might "need" to make your life "good."

18. At open-bar events, start by tipping the bartender(s) $20. They should take care of you the rest of the night. Let them know you respect and acknowledge them, because they're your dance-juice gatekeepers.

19. Google that rash. Or don't Google it. Sometimes living in blissful ignorance is equally fun as applying a topical ointment.

20. Chips and salsa are a perfectly respectable adult meal. Also, chips and salsa are great to have in your house for expected and unexpected guests. Who doesn't like chips and salsa? Vegans and meat-chewers alike can finally find common ground.

21. When adding someone to your contacts, write something specific. For example: Joe Interesting Wedding Dancer, Megan Lopsided Hair, Chris Red Lobster Adonis.

22. Crest Whitestrips actually work. (Not sponsored. But I WISH.)

23. Succulents make the perfect gift. A box of succulents make for a super-quick/cheap/seemingly cultured gift. You can give them to a man or a woman and they're easy to keep alive. Trust me, I kill everything (that's legal to kill).

24. You can never have too many tampons. Put them in any and every bag you might carry. Guys and gals alike, many a vagina will thank you.

25. Have easy-to-prepare food in the house at all times. This is essential. Your drunk and/or tired self will be so, so grateful.

26. The dogs of the Internet make it better. The dogs on Instagram in particular are an AMAZING resource for consoling people who are sad. Don't worry if you don't know what to say to that friend who just got dumped—send her the link to @beanzhart on Instagram and her day will turn around. If she doesn't derive any happiness from that dog, then she needs to do some digging and find out why she's terrible.

27. It's okay if you don't know how to pronounce that

thing on the menu. If you don't know how to say the name of that entrée or wine, just tell the server you want their best pee-knot greg-eyo. And then give them two thumbs down with a smile and tell them to figure that out.

28. **Always tip the valet.** So much can be learned about a person based on the inside of their car. I currently have two empty bags of rice cakes, some old dried-up makeup wipes, and a variety of dirty gym clothes in my car. The valet that has to spend time in that mess deserves at least a five.

29. **The car wash is a great place to be alone.** You can gather your thoughts to the soothing sound of rubber slapping glass. Also, it's nice to wash your car from time to time.

30. **Have clothing and accessories specifically dedicated to rain.** Uggs are not rain boots. Umbrellas are cool.

31. **You're not terrible because you didn't bring a reusable bag to the grocery store.** Yes, everyone else that did is clearly better than you, but you're not the worst. Just try to recycle in other areas of your life to balance it out.

32. **Salt, pepper, Tabasco sauce, and ranch dressing are the only condiments you need.**

33. **You don't need that gross underwear anymore.** I know you rationalize it as "that time of the month" underwear, but that time of the month doesn't happen all month, so treat yourself. Your privates deserve something nice.

34. **Wash your dishes.** Your sink can be a reflection of your state of mind. If I'm having a tough day or a difficult time, I find washing dishes makes me feel better. When my sink is clean, my brain feels clear.

35. **Moist towelettes can be a real lifesaver.** You never know when you're going to be held up at gunpoint and forced to stick your arms in jelly.

36. **Portable speakers make showers more fun!**

37. **Tip the hotel housekeeping.** They know ALL your secrets. WOOF.

38. **Find a good hairstylist.** Getting your hair done, especially for a lady, can be an awkward, annoying task. It usually takes a long time, you're going to have to have an extended conversation, and if you don't like what they did there can be problems. Once you find that person who nails your look, like a romantic relationship, hold on tight!

39. **One wallet is all you need.** Ladies, you can have a ton of purses but try to only have one wallet. As a serial purse and wallet swapper, I lose so many important things in the switch. So try to keep your money, IDs, credit cards, and ever-important loyalty cards in one place.

40. **Buy a few stain sticks and put them in strategic places.** Your bathroom, your car, your bag, your kitchen, etc.

41. **Work on your handshake.** It says a lot about you as a person and you can't redo it once it's done. Unless that becomes your handshake—the twice-over. Interesting choice.

42. **Don't wear a shirt with a band/ musical artist on it.** Unless you're ready to have conversations with strangers about it.

43. **Keep extra blankets and pillows in your house.** It's very classy to actually have clean bedding for your guests.

44. **Have a "guest basket" of toiletries.** This will make you seem like a WONDERFULLY THOUGHTFUL person. I know because I've been the guest in a house that had this type of basket, and I immediately felt like I should give them my first child.

45. **If you can't find the expiration date, don't eat it.** It's not worth the potential diarrhea at the office.

46. **Never FORCE someone to watch/ look at/read your creative project/work/ game.** Think about whether they really want to offer their opinion before you make them do it.

47. **Don't hold a grudge.** Especially over a board game. Do you really want the news headline "Board Game Becomes Sword Maim" written about you?

48. **Use Q-tips sometimes!**

49. **Invest in a giant Costco-sized bottle of pain medicine.** It's worth it.

50. **Be nice.**

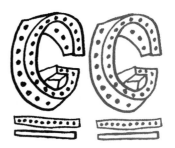

THE ART OF FAKING IT UNTIL SOMEONE CALLS YOU OUT ON IT

THE ART OF DOING THE LEAST
TO GET PAID MORE
THAN YOU DID FOR BABYSITTING

THE ART OF FINDING YOUR INNER PANTS SUIT
AND YOUR OUTER SWEATPANTS

The Art of Balance, Commitment, and Finding the Bathroom No One Else Uses

THE ART OF CONVINCING A STRANGER TO GIVE
YOU MONEY FOR USING A COMPUTER

THE ART OF MINIMIZING YOUR DEBT
AND MAXIMIZING YOUR POTENTIAL
TO LEARN WHAT THE WORD
"COLLATE" MEANS

THE ART OF EXPANDING YOUR MIND AND DEBT

THE ART OF HOPEFULLY, EVENTUALLY MAKING
SOME MONEY FOR DOING A JOB RELATIVELY CLOSE
TO SOMETHING YOU SORT OF ENJOY

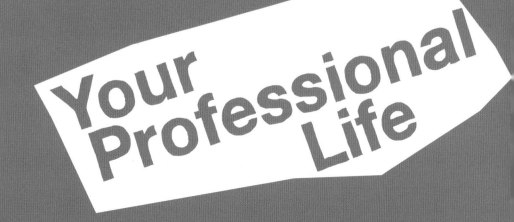

Your
Professional
Life

I can practically smell the blazers and the classy leather business side-satchels.

Welcome to the part of the book about school and your brain and your professional life. I can practically smell the blazers and the classy leather business side-satchels.

When I was a little girl I used to flip through JCPenney's giant annual holiday catalog and **circle all the toys I wanted** for Christmas that year. I remember circling things like the cash register set; the "little miss professional" attaché case, complete with a giant fake cell phone and legal pad; the nurse play set; the pop-up chalkboard; you get the idea. My favorite toys were all business/work-related. I was already an entrepreneur and I hadn't even finished second grade.

Of course, I wanted dolls and princess dress-up kits, too, but my dad didn't like Barbie and the female ideal she represented. The only Barbie he ever caved and bought me was Native American Barbie, because he thought it had educational value. What a guy. He loves education and hard work. I remember in fifth grade, I had an assignment to try to re-create something associated with the Sioux Indians. My dad and I set out to make a papoose. What I mean by that is my dad made a papoose. A papoose is a cradle backpack that the Native Americans used to carry their children. They looked something like this:

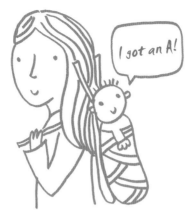

I ~~watched~~ helped my dad gather sticks, glue them together onto a piece of wood and tie them off with brown suede rope, then hand-stitch burlap into the shape of a headpiece, and decorate the entire structure with beads and feathers. I had to stop him before he tried to put a fake baby inside for "realism." When I brought in my project, it was clear that I hadn't made it. Everyone else brought in handmade bows and arrows or rocks that they had painted with native motifs. I had a life-sized papoose. My dad got an A.

His feverish passion for work and education really influenced me as I got older. I became a sort of nerd-jock hybrid in high school. I always wanted to get good grades, I always wanted to win my events at track meets, I performed in plays, and I joined all the clubs I thought I should join to make my résumé look appealing to colleges. I even competed in mock trial for one year, until I realized that I'm NOT a good lawyer. I just liked the excuse to wear a lady suit.

By the time I was a senior, the effort paid off. I got a full ride to the first college I applied to. Granted, it was a small liberal arts college in northern New Jersey that had an alarming number of skunks running around the campus (like, actual skunks; they were not in the brochure). But they took me on early decision in December and

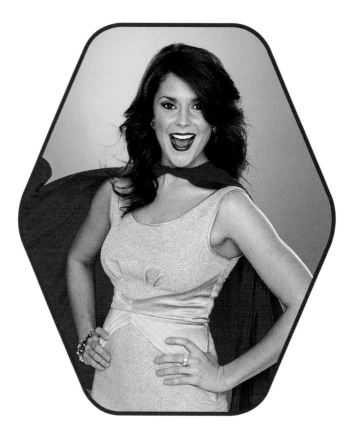

I thought, *Well, okay, I guess my college-search thing is done, cool.* While everyone else sent out all of their applications and did campus visits and interviews, I was done. It felt great.

Until I got there. I had a *terrible* time adjusting. Turns out I hate change and I'm not good at socializing. Good to know! I got really depressed and sat in my room a lot, researching other colleges. At one point, I started filling out applications to other, bigger schools like NYU and UCLA, because I thought they'd give me a more "authentic" college experience. Our college didn't have a football team and our mascot was the road runner (NOT the cartoon character) and there were skunks all over and I had ten Bulgarian exchange students living on my floor—this was not a real school.

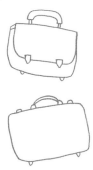

But then I had a conversation with my mom and she encouraged me to stick it out until the end of the semester to see if I could find just one thing I liked. After all, it was a free ride, and it was up to me to make the most of it. So I did what I do best: I worked hard. I got a job off campus, I signed up for indoor track (turns out I had lost my edge and was no longer competitive in track—also fun to learn!), and I made friends with the Bulgarians, who turned out to be some of the nicest, most hilarious people.

Eventually over the next few years I found my niche. I got into writing and performing and started interning in the city while working two off-campus jobs (you'll hear all about it) and I finally started to sort of enjoy my experience. For a while after I graduated, I still lived in regret that I missed out on a super-fun college experience. But as I got more involved in the professional world, I became grateful for the experience. Also, the lack of college loans is a very nice thing. I'm still not the most social person in the world (I work on the Internet), nor am I the smartest in the brain department (no doy), but I do know how to put hard work into something. So welcome to the part of the book where I try to give you guidance whether you're still in school or making the leap into the professional world.

The most helpful advice I can give you is to work hard. Take it or leave it. But if you leave it, make sure you recycle it—don't litter. There's a tip!

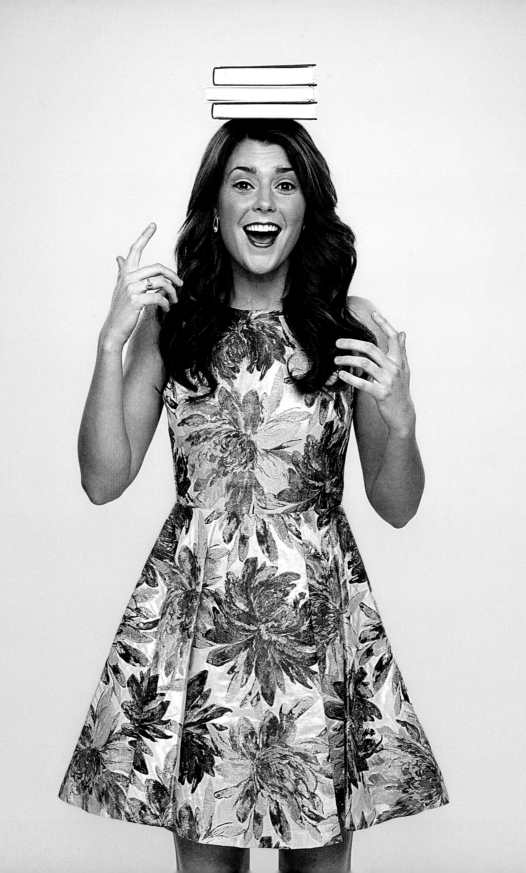

HOW TO
BALANCE WORK AND PLAY

I'm a notorious workaholic. It's something my dad unintentionally taught me. He used to come to my high school track meets, and right after I'd clear a high jump I'd look over and he'd be furiously working on land-planning blueprints or writing his presentations for building developments or whatever it is he does. I tell everyone he's a professional planner. He has one of those tall drafting tables and collects soil samples (aka bags of dirt) from areas people want to build on. That's really all I know about what he does for a living. I should probably ask him more about it. Dad was always working and he was great at it, but I'm not sure if he totally loved his job.

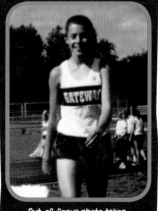
Out-of-focus photo taken by my dad at a track meet.

Following in his footsteps, I accidentally got really into working. Having multiple jobs became one of my special skills. I've had almost every crappy job imaginable in retail and food service. My first job was as a fitting room attendant at T.J.Maxx. But after I spent a month there watching SO MANY middle-aged women blatantly try to steal clothes by hiding them under their own clothes, Chili's called looking for a hostess, and they paid fifty cents more an hour. BOOM. Upgrade.

When I went to college, I used working as a way to avoid socializing. Yay! I started my freshman year as a server at Chili's. I had finally graduated from being a hostess to being a server—a dream come true.

One summer, I took things to an extreme. I had a job working at an Applebee's in Hamilton, New Jersey, near my dad's house three days a week, and a second job at a Dave & Buster's working another three days a week in Philadelphia near my mom's house. On my day off, I'd go visit my boyfriend in Central Jersey. That summer, I specialized in driving across New Jersey and being tired. Dave & Buster's kitchen staff was comprised of rehabilitated criminals, and after every shift a security guard had to escort me to my car. It was all very glamorous.

Of course, I was miserable and eventually I cracked from exhaustion . . . in the middle of a Target parking lot. I was leaving the store after shopping with my mom and I became hysterical in the parking lot at just the thought of going to my dinner shift later that afternoon. My mom was so disturbed by my deteriorating mental state that she made me quit on the spot. I called and cried and quit. You would think that I'd have learned my lesson then about balancing work and play and not overcommitting myself based on this experience, but no.

When I was a junior in college, I upped the ante. I taught tennis on the weekends in addition to working the Thursday and Friday night shifts at Applebee's. By "teaching tennis" I really mean: throwing tennis balls at upper-middle-class kids whose parents wanted one hour to drink Chardonnay alone. On top of Applebee's and teaching tennis, I arranged my schedule so that I only had classes two days a week and added internships to the mix. I was technically only required to do one internship in order to get my degree in communications. HOWEVER, because I was addicted to working and desperate to set myself up for success post-college, every semester I made a copy of the internship form for the workplace advisor to sign, so that I could apply for a new internship—without raising any eyebrows or getting approval by the school. By the time I graduated, I'd had five internships. I only got college credit for the first one. I was making copies and getting coffee for my twentysomething bosses without any compensation—credit or otherwise. This was technically illegal.

After I graduated, it seemed like all that hustling (and not having fun) was for nothing. I moved in with the guy I was dating (who was still in school and living with four other boys) and I worked at the local Olive Garden. There I learned that people can shovel an incredible amount of carbs down their throats when endless pasta bowls are promised. I saw a lot of overeating that can't be unseen.

Two months into my Olive Garden experience I got a call from one of my internship advisors offering me a job. COLLEGE WAS WORTH IT! Essentially, the company I interned for over three separate semesters created a position for me so they could feel less guilty about using all of my time for free. Also, I like to think that I was relatively competent. That's debatable, but back then I was sharp(er) and quiet and desperate.

Meanwhile, I had just moved into a Brooklyn apartment with my college roommate that was an hour train ride away from my job in Manhattan. Every morning, I woke up and took the train and got to work and did about two hours of real work over the course of an eight-hour workday, and then took the train home to shoot vlogs with my roommate or attend an improv class in the city. In between "work-work," I'd work on comedy sketches and screenplays when my boss wasn't looking at my computer. We shared an office—woof.

My boss was amazing. She was probably ten years older than me, the former president of her college sorority, an incredible project manager who could balance work and play like I've never seen. She could organize a fifty-person commercial shoot, a charity 5K for her sorority, and her own wedding at the same time. And then at the end of the day she'd hit up a happy hour with friends for two hours and head back to her house in Jersey. She was great. She inadvertently taught me so much about organization and time management and personal enjoyment. I was really bad at all three, especially the personal enjoyment part.

After about four months of working at that company, I came to the conclusion that I wanted to pursue comedy full-time. I quit and found a job with more flexible hours at a restaurant called Houston's (essentially an upmarket Chili's in the middle of Manhattan). Three months and a few dropped rib platters later, I got the opportunity to start my professional Internet-video-making adventure. I was hired by a website and I got to work from home, which was A DREAM COME TRUE. I had no boss looking at my computer, no table I had to tell the specials to, and no

spoiled kids with clothes that cost more than my car that I had to throw tennis balls at. It was just me, myself, and I(nternet). With that, I very quickly learned that it was up to me to manage my time and keep myself on a schedule that both got my work done and allowed me to have fun.

After seeing my dad quietly labor over a job he never enjoyed that much, my only aspiration as an adult was to get paid to do something I love. And, OMG, it's happening. And I want to keep it happening. But I do believe that "all work and no play makes Grace a dull girl," so setting aside and enjoying plenty of downtime is something I'm working on.

Here are some of my thoughts on how you can balance work and play. Because life is cool when it's cool.

Incentivize

Treat yo'self.

Give yourself something to look forward to if you get *x* amount of work done. When I was a kid, my mom had a whole star-sticker system. If we did our chores that week we'd get a star sticker, if we were well behaved we'd get a star sticker. At the end of the week we'd be rewarded according to however many star stickers we had collected. This might be why I'm very competitive as an adult.

In kindergarten, I remember we were rewarded via a similar system, and at the end of each week the two students with the highest behavior ratings got to have a McDonald's lunch with the teacher. MCDONALD'S. Remember how those women in Oprah's audience reacted when she told them they were each getting a free car? That was me the week I got to have the McDonald's lunch. I was freaking the F out. And, even at five years old, I really felt like I'd earned

it. I consciously worked on folding my hands in my lap and hanging up my coat and putting the foam blocks away.

And as an adult I try to give myself incentives to get my work done, too. Weirdly, it's mostly still McDonald's. And vodka and Forever 21.

Group Accountability

Peer pressure. The good kind.

When I really want to get work done I find it's helpful to tell my friends and/or strangers about what I want to accomplish. This creates group/ social accountability. Good friends make each other feel guilty for not doing the work they've committed to finishing. It's also pretty inspiring to talk to your friends about the things they want to accomplish in the next few weeks/months/years.

Look Up Inspirational People

Nothing is more inspiring than a six-year-old prodigy. The other day my friend Mamrie and I were independently working on projects and each took a break

child prodigy
child prodigy
child prodigy piano
child prodigy painter
child prodigy music

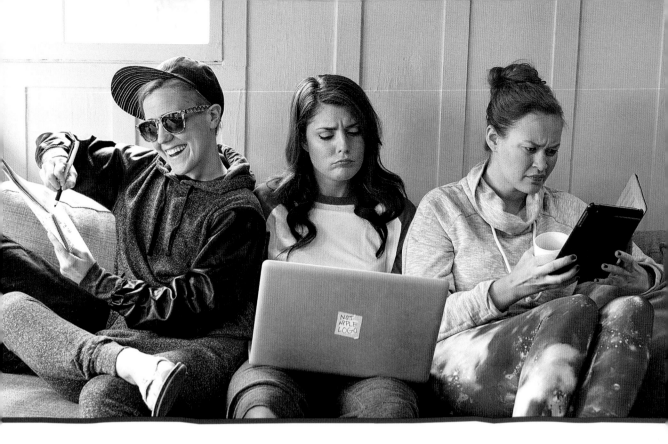

to watch an adorable apartment tour video on YouTube from a very beautiful, completely put-together beauty guru. Why? Because we both know she's better at life than us and we wanted to be inspired. Granted, immediately afterward Mamrie ordered six candles off Amazon and I took a shot of vodka, but it worked. We were both reinspired to be better, more productive people.

I highly recommend looking up child prodigies and/or any individual you believe is doing life better than you. This is the sole reason Pinterest exists.

Organize

Make a list.

Simply writing out what you need to get done can help you cross things off the list. This is such an obvious tip, but something I forget to do, and it helps. Just like showering. It gives you a visual so you can prioritize (it's the Jazzercise of organizing). Prioritizing saves time. Also, please remind me to shower. Adding to the list.

Out

Get outta there.

When work is done, or when you feel a lull in your creative energy, change up your environment. Get out of your traditional workspace. Get off of work email and check in with friends and family. Give your brain a new setting to buzz around and have fun/relax in. If you ate bread every meal for days at a time and then ate pizza, your body would be all like, *WTF, YAAAAAS.* It'd be stimulating and exciting and delicious. Also,

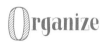

get out and do something that isn't work-related. Hike, exercise, sleep, laser tag, hit a piñata, dump some dinner rolls down a hill, have fun, whatever. Also, going out and doing social stuff is very good for your soul, apparently. See: other self-help books.

Drugs

Don't do them.
Be cool, dude.

Ambience

Seduce yourself.
One of the best ways to get work done is to create an inspiring, comfortable environment. What makes you feel relaxed? What makes you feel stimulated? Candles? Music? A photo of Jonathan Taylor Thomas? I'm just spit-balling. I have some friends that decorate their space with vision boards (or, as I like to call them, adorable adult collages) to give them inspiration. My mom likes to have motivational quotes around her and occasionally she makes me listen to the audio version of *The Secret*, because it has soothing gong noises in between each chapter.

Personally, when I work, I like complete silence or I listen to one song on repeat. At the moment my go-to is Billy Joel's "We Didn't Start the Fire," because it's powerful and for some reason makes me feel like I'm doing a complicated, beautiful ice-skating routine. Otherwise, I like having access to chips nearby and a solo bathroom while I work. Very professional.

Wager

Your best bet is against yourself.
Turn your work into a tiny, personal casino. This isn't for everyone, but sometimes I find I get more work done when I bet against myself. I make a silent, private wager that I won't get a certain amount of stuff done, but if I do, I win! What do I win? It ranges, from clothing to an episode of *Real Housewives* to a meal at The Cheesecake Factory (I am a champion!). This is very similar to the incentivize step, except more self-shaming if you don't win. If it helps and encourages you, try betting a friend. Combine the incentive and group accountability steps and raise the stakes. Designate rewards and punishments (within reason, you sadomasochist). See what happens. If it ends up being detrimental, then maybe don't do it again.

Good Job

You did something!
Take a second to congratulate yourself on accomplishing something. There are a lot of people in this world who do nothing. Trust me, I see them in my mirror when I'm very hungover. You did something! You should be proud. Cool job doing life, stranger. Take a vacation! I'm happy for you. Unless the thing you did was criminal or not helpful to your mental health or to our society as a whole, then I say stop it.

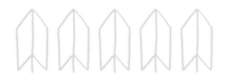

Ideas for personal incentives if you get x amount of work done:

- A dog.
- A really kewl dessert.
- Some trash TV.
- Online clothes shopping.
- Chinese food.
- Two dogs.

Ideas for inspiring things to look up online:

- Child prodigies.
- YouTube beauty gurus.
- Beyoncé.
- A montage of someone on a weight-loss show losing weight and gaining confidence.
- Beyoncé.
- A documentary about Kenyan marathon runners.
- Beyoncé.

Remember:

IGLOO DAWG

Incentivize

Group Accountability

Look Up Inspirational People

Organize

Out

Drugs

Ambience

Wager

Good Job

#IGLOODAWG

HOW TO BALANCE WORK AND PLAY

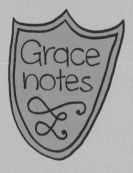

☐   What are your short-term goals (for the next year)?

_____

☐   What are your long-term goals (after this year)?

_____

☐   How long has it been since you've taken a vacation?

_____

☐   What was the last "fun" thing you did? (And no, taxes aren't fun.)

_____

☐   What was the last "successful professional" thing you did? (And no, having sex with a college professor isn't a suc-sex-ful professor-nal thing.)

_____

☐   How long has it been since you've talked to:

Your significant other?   _____

Your parental figure?   _____

Your best friend?   _____

That medium-sized unknown animal you sometimes talk to late at night?

_____

☐   What's your emotional state right now?

_____

WELL, HEY, you filled out this worksheet! That's something! **HIGH-FIVE!**

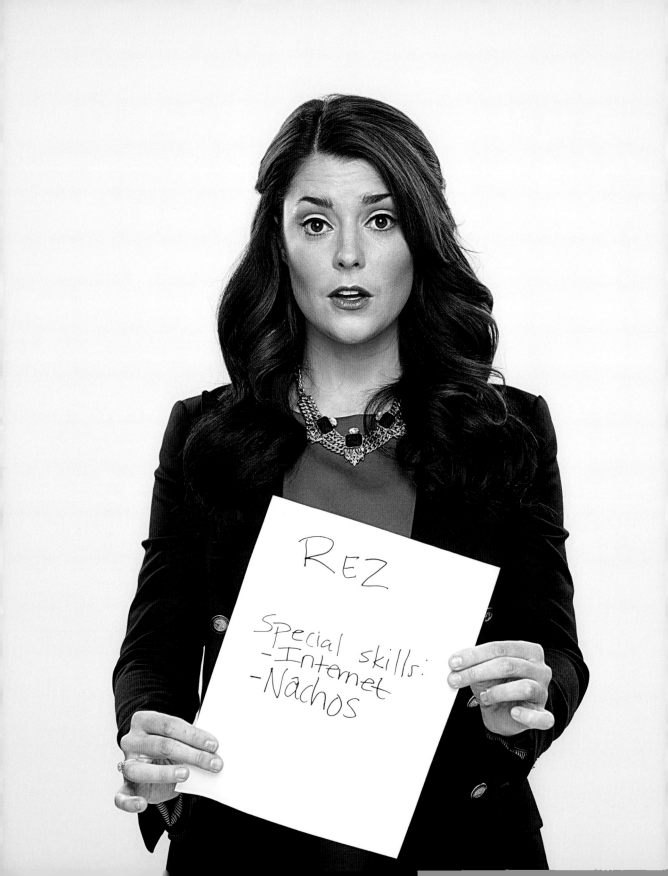

HOW TO
INTERVIEW
FOR
A
JOB

I've interviewed for my fair share of jobs. Like Pokémon cards, I've collected an assortment of chain restaurants on my résumé. So far I've got Chili's, Applebee's, Dave & Buster's, Olive Garden, Houston's, and Sails (a short-lived pretentious Jersey Shore restaurant on the bay). Yet despite having all of that experience, somehow I didn't get hired for the NBC Page Program.

For those of you who don't know, the NBC Page Program (think Kenneth on *30 Rock*) is essentially a paid internship at NBC. It's very "prestigious" and "illustrious" and "reputable." After a semester interning at *Late Night with Conan O'Brien*, I got an opportunity to interview for a coveted spot in the program. This was going to be my first real foray into a professional world that didn't include mozzarella sticks. This was

my ticket! Once I made it into the program, I was sure that some higher-up at NBC would just happen to see me in the hallway and think I was so off-the-cuff hilarious that he'd offer me my own show on the spot. THIS WAS MY CHANCE! What would I call my show? *Grace's Company? Grace Expectations? Grace Helbig and Ellen DeGeneres Are Best Friends Forever?*

The interview did not work out as planned.

I was SO nervous. My armpits decided to do their best impression of Slip 'n Slides as I verbally farted my way through the interview. At this point in my life, I thought the interviewer held my whole future in her hands. Except her hands were busy. She was instant-messaging the entire time. I could see the reflection of her computer screen in the window behind her. Occasionally, I

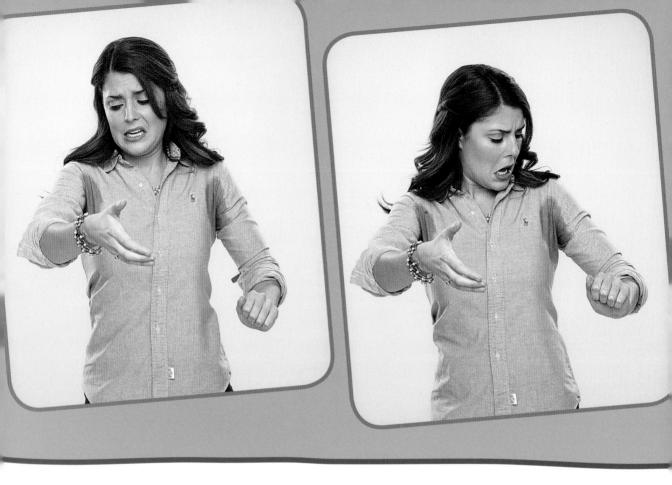

thought she was laughing at my witty anecdotes, but no. Whoever she was messaging with was HILARIOUS.

The worst part is that I spent so long that morning trying to iron my only pair of "business pants" on my teeny-tiny space-saving dorm room ironing board while imagining what sort of antics I'd work into my *SNL* opening monologue. I didn't get the job. Ultimately, it was for the best. The page uniform is a blazer and pencil skirt. I look like an uncomfortable teen mom/PTA member in a pencil skirt. Sigh. I'M NOT BITTER.

I've had time to reflect on past job interviews, assess (ASS!) my performance, pick out my strengths and weaknesses, and now I feel much more knowledgeable on the subject. Which is

why I feel comfortable writing this chapter—that, and I'm writing it in sweatpants and not a GOD-DAMN PENCIL SKIRT. Look at me now, baby!

ant

Want it.

Even if it sucks socks and is strictly a survival job, ACT LIKE YOU WANT IT! Odds are that your unadulterated passion for the job will inspire confidence—or the interviewer will find you completely annoying. Life is a highway. And if this is a legit life-changing opportunity, don't be afraid to express your DESIRE for it. It's just like my desire to eat chips for breakfast or my desire to see tiny dogs in human clothes. I REALLY

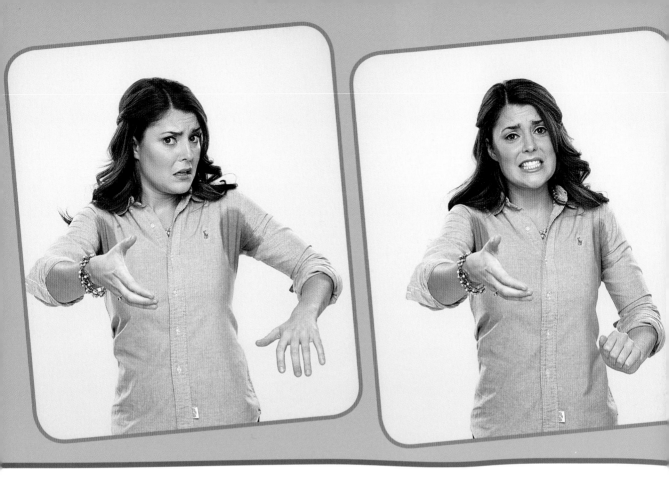

WANT THOSE THINGS. And I'm not afraid to let that influence my actions; I'm not allowed in three or four Petcos in both New York and California. That's beside the point.

Passion and a positive attitude are key.

Organize

Get it together.
Organize your résumé and your social media.

Yes, writing a résumé seems SO STUPID. But then again, your potential boss could just look at your Facebook page and realize one of your special skills is drinking Bacardi and Diet Cokes out of curly, sparkly straws. So organize a piece of paper that proves otherwise. And also organize a

PRIVATE Facebook album for all of those photos. Yes, the ones with the pancakes. You're a freak, but you're excellent at data entry, so make sure that's what they see.

Research

Google that creature.
Find out your interviewer's name and let Google do the work. Is he interested in baseball? Whoa! All of a sudden you mention the Dodgers offhand. OOPS. Does she love *Breaking Bad*? Oh my god, suddenly a clear blue meth metaphor sneaks its way into your spiel about how pure your love is for what you do. DOUBLE OOPS. Use the Internet to your advantage on this one. BUT

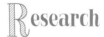

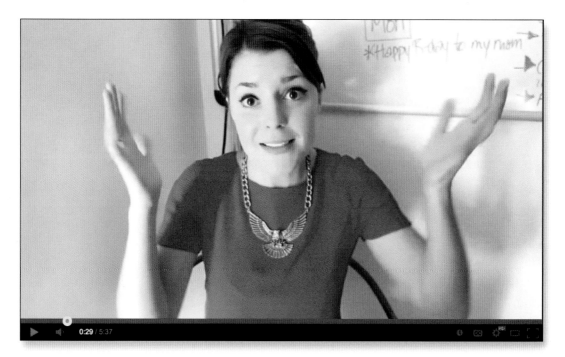

DON'T BE A WEIRDO. Remember: treat Internet "strangers" the way you'd want Internet "strangers" to treat you.

Klean

Rinse off your person.

Clean isn't spelled with a *k*, but you don't have a job, so shut up. Wash your junk, iron your clothes, wear deodorant, and brush your hair. Everything else is a bonus.

Prep

Wrap your mind around it.

Try to predict the questions you'll be asked and familiarize yourself with the company, so that you can ask smart questions about the job. You've seen enough TV and movies with interview scenes. Those "fictitious" questions they're asking ARE REAL QUESTIONS. Go online and Google "standard interview questions." They might ask you about your strengths, they might ask you about your weaknesses, they might ask you about the fake job you made up on your résumé listing your BFF as the manager. Have an answer prepared—anything, just be ready. You are your own Miss America contestant in this moment. So don't be Miss South Carolina. OLD REFERENCE, GOOGLE IT.

Original

You are the only version of you, unless you're a twin. Ew.

When prepping your answers, remember not to be a generic piece of bread. Bread isn't delicious, but bread BOWLS are. Yes, I do realize that most of my metaphors are food-related; it's a choice. Do you have a mouth? Oh good, then you can relate.

Make your answers UNIQUE. Different is good. You don't want to be hired somewhere because you're a sheep. It'd be weird for T.J.Maxx to hire

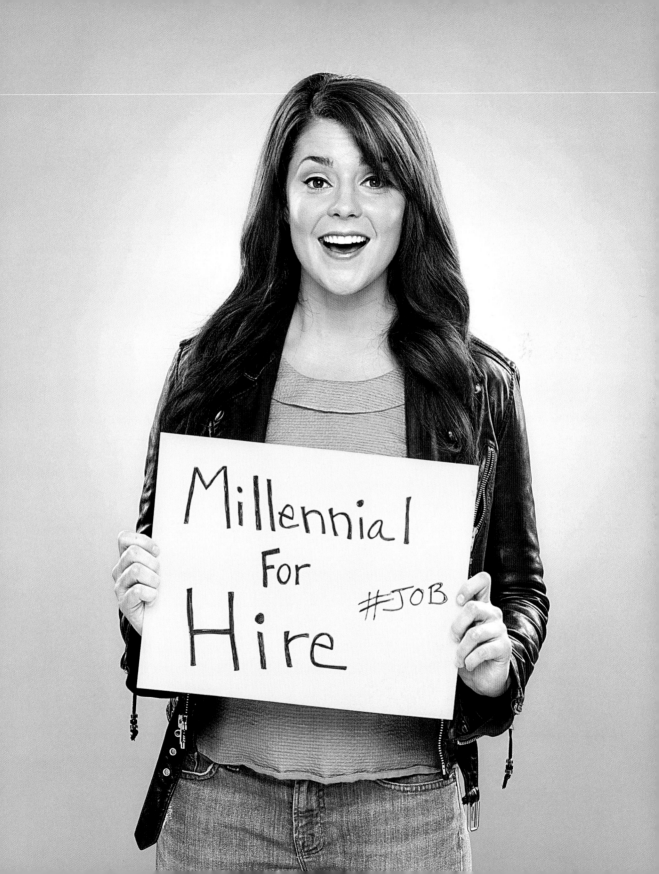

Talk Back

Follow up.

Talk back to your interviewer. Not like that. Don't be a sass ass. Talk back as in follow up after the interview. I like to find one specific, personal thing we might have talked about in the meeting to lead off my email. For instance, "Hey, Jeff, glad to know you have such strong opinions on popsicles, too. Anyway, it was great meeting you and I hope we can find some way to work together in the future." Make sure to send this email maybe one to five days after your original meeting so you don't seem too aggressive/ too already forgettable.

a sheep to run their fitting room. Yes, they'd get at least one viral video out of it, but that sheep would have a very hard time moving up the corporate ladder. Make sure that the company hires YOU.

On Time

Get there.

Just do it. JUST. DO. IT. This is your future boss's first impression of you and if you're late, he's going to think, *Well, this person must do drugs*, or *This person must have had to go to the abortion clinic this morning*, or *This person must have had to appear on* The Maury Povich Show *this morning to find out if he IS IN FACT the father*. Who knows? Minds wander.

I like to schedule meetings in my calendar a half hour earlier than they actually are, because I know I'm a chronically late person and this is a fun way to trick myself!

QUICK REMINDERS

- Like old bread, **MOLD** these tips to work for your specific interview.
- If you don't get the job, **WHO CARES?** Except your parents and your bank account and your real/fake significant other, and your future. Interviews are good practice.
- As long as you didn't visibly piss or poop yourself, it was a **GREAT** interview. Move on.

Remember: 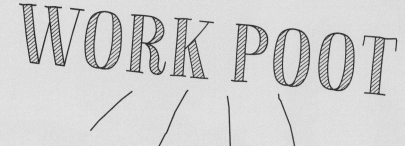 **WORK POOT**

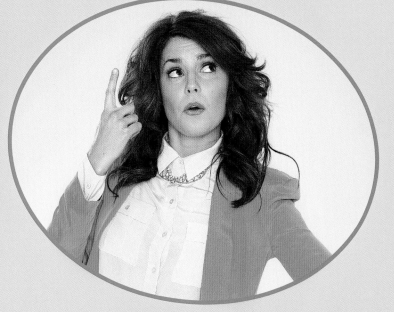

Want   **P**rep

Organize   **O**riginal

Research   **O**n Time

Klean   **T**alk Back

#WORKPOOT

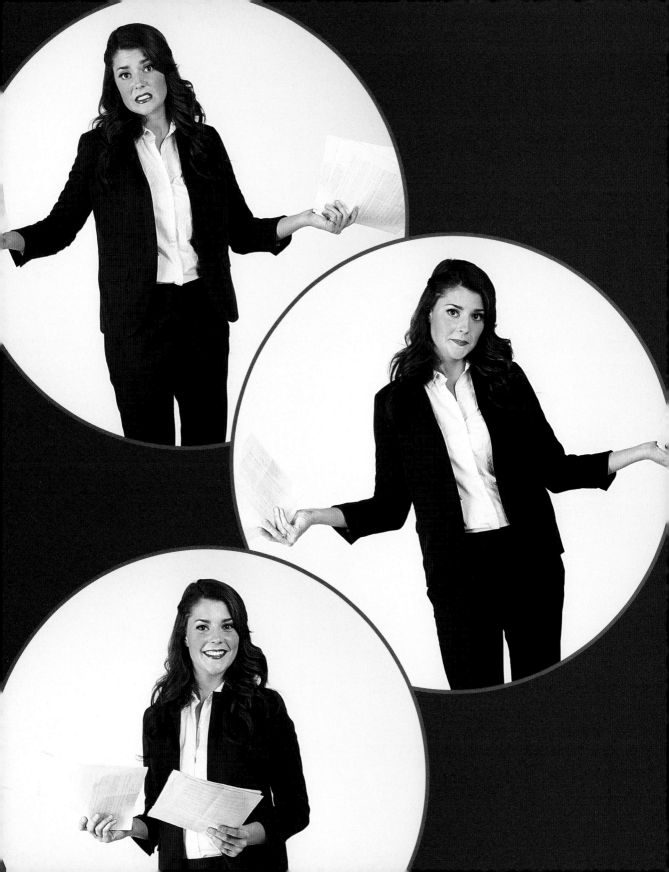

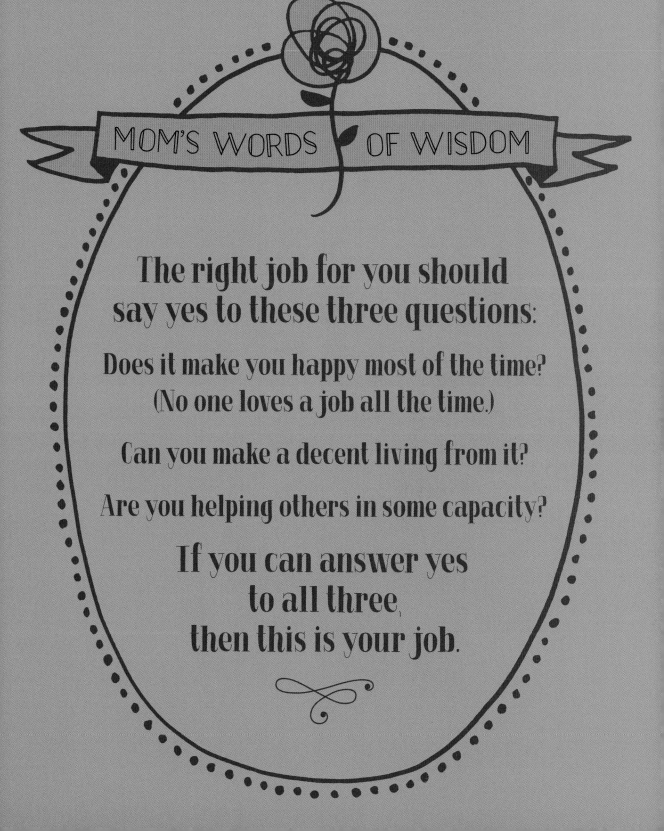

MOM'S WORDS OF WISDOM

The right job for you should
say yes to these three questions:

Does it make you happy most of the time?
(No one loves a job all the time.)

Can you make a decent living from it?

Are you helping others in some capacity?

If you can answer yes
to all three,
then this is your job.

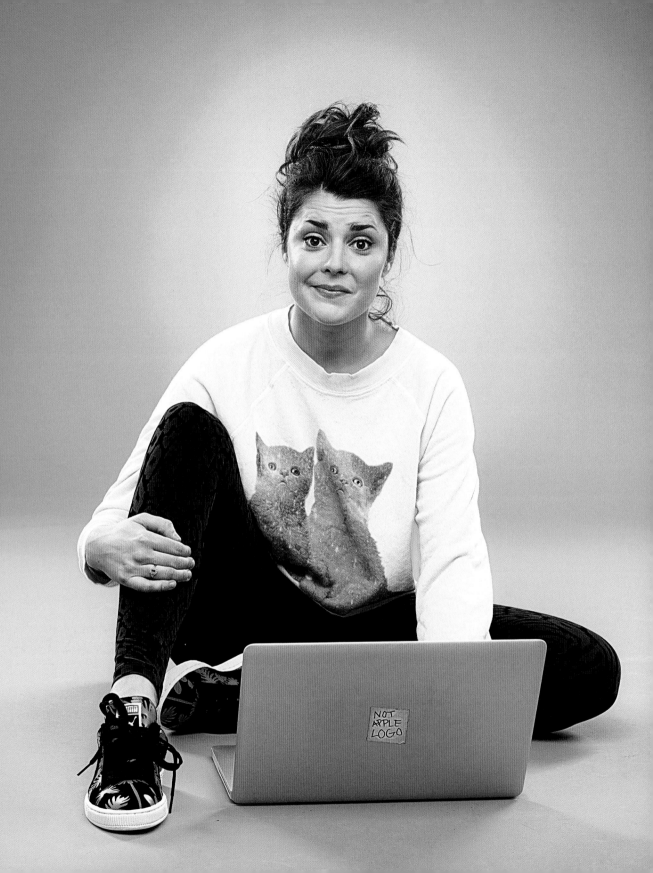

TIPS
FOR SURVIVING IN SCHOOL AND IN THE OFFICE

School can be depressing when you realize it's where you've spent most of your youth. Same thing for time spent in the office, which will likely stretch to include most of your adult life. Ack! Unless you like your job. Then great job! Literally.

I went to high school. I even went to college. Hard to believe, I know. I currently make a living talking by myself to a camera while putting condiments on my face and emoting about Miley Cyrus's crotch. I'm using my degree to the fullest.

Your academic career can be both the greatest and the absolute worst time of your life. It can be wonderful, because you have a safety net to experiment and be dumb. But it can also be miserable, because it's one of the most transitional times in your life and no one gives you a guidebook to figure it out. EXCEPT FOR ME! Sort

of. Not really; you're going to have very harsh personal experiences that I could never prepare you for. ZOIKS!

I did five internships in college—all in office settings. And after college I had an office job. I got a company email address, I went to a store and bought three pairs of "work pants," and I tried to actually iron my clothes in the morning. It was uncomfortable. On top of that, I'm convinced that fluorescent lights were invented by an evil, reincarnated epileptic with a vendetta. THERE'S ALWAYS ONE FLICKERING AND AS SOON AS YOU LOOK AT IT, IT STOPS. After four(ish) months, I couldn't handle it anymore and I quit.

Surviving in an office job is similar to surviving in school. When you're first trying to adapt, you don't know if you'll ever find your place, but eventually your new friend Chyle (with a "Ch") convinces you to stick it out. Here are twenty tips for school and twenty for work.

Remember that by having a job or going to school you're doing something positive for yourself—that is, unless you're just doing it because of intense pressure from family members. Yay!

SCHOOL

1. **Don't go after the hottest person.** They're probably overcompensating for something terrible hidden underneath all that pretty hair.

2. **Get at least 80 percent of your homework done the night before.** College life is almost entirely about 80 percent prep work and 20 percent spontaneous problem-solving/improvising.

3. **Lump yourself with like-minded people.** In an academic environment it's easier to be successful if you're surrounded and inspired by people who "get" you and vice versa. When I was in college, I found a group of friends who liked comedy and we created a sketch comedy TV show for our campus TV network and performed episodic improv shows every Monday night. Looking back, I realize it was pretty terrible, but at the time it gave me confidence to pursue comedy after I graduated. Cool!

4. **Try to get your housing figured out early.** This can be one of the most stressful parts about college. Figure out who you want to live with next year and where, so you're not an anxious puddle of tears in a windowless room with the girl who sleep-screams.

5. **You don't *really* need to know math.** Unless you're majoring in it or are a professional human calculator.

6. **Don't make fun of nerds.** Just don't. Eventually, they're going to dominate you and/or strategize a twenty-five-year-long brilliant slow burn prank on you and your loved ones. They'll get the last, wheezy laugh.

7. **Keep all of your important things in one bag.** This is also overall life advice. Leaving something important in a classroom or someone else's dorm is annoying. You *just* finished your walk of shame, don't make yourself have to go back. Keep it together.

8. **Don't be the teacher's pet.**

9. **Experiment. Sexually.** Only if you're in college. Get it out of your system now, because orgies are frowned upon in the workplace.

10. **Be social.** Push yourself to mingle with other social groups. This allows "friendships" to happen. Whoa! Neat!

11. **Look, everyone has student loans. Don't complain.**

12. **If you're a lady, it's super cool to carry some sort of spray poison in case of on-campus crazies.** In fact, I encourage carrying both wonderful-smelling body splash/perfume

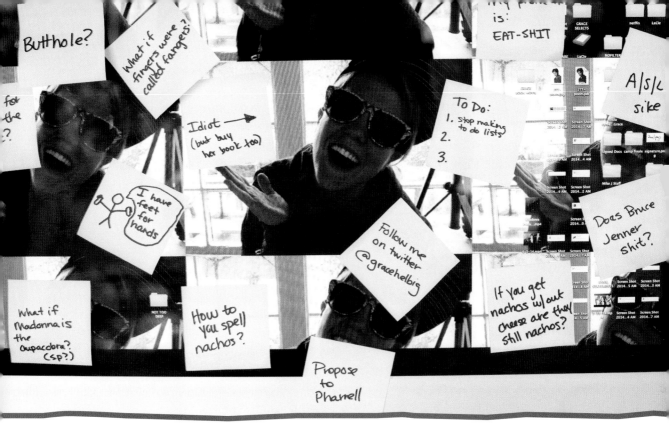

along with eye-burning spray toxins. I currently own Mace, bear spray, and Cold Steel Inferno pepper spray. (Side note: Google-search "Cold Steel" and treat yourself to a night of amazing video commercials for self-defense weapons sold by a slightly overweight, middle-aged man named Lynn.)

13. When in doubt, refer to your syllabus.

14. Don't get on the bad side of the sad person who lives on your dorm floor. Respect them and assume they could kill you at any moment, so be nice ☺!

15. Make a mental map of all of the cleanest, least popular public bathrooms on campus. Living in New York and having to be out of my apartment for most of the day going from an audition to a meeting to a rehearsal, I started to make a mental map of all the most accessible and most private public bathrooms where I could change clothes, fix my face, and/or empty my bladder, etc., if necessary. (Urban city note: Hotel bathrooms are great. If you walk into a hotel with confidence, they'll assume you're a guest and not a stranger off the street hoping to take a private dump.)

16. Colleges that have radio ads probably aren't the best colleges. That said, my college had a radio ad.

17. Shower shoes are a great investment.

18. Maybe stay away from the person with cold sores.

19. You can get so many tampons and condoms for free from your health center. Take advantage.

20. If you hate it, it won't last forever.

WORK

1. Try to avoid office romances. Office crushes are SO FUN, but don't blur lines. Sorry, Robin Thicke.

2. Experiment. Professionally. If you're a science major, please take this tip literally. Otherwise, if you're a student or young professional, take the time to test different occupations and see what clicks.

3. Network! Pack the ChapStick, because networking is the ass-kissing professional socialization that happens when you hang out with people in similar fields who all want to advance. But don't force the networking; try to let it happen organically. Like dry-humping at the end of a first date.

4. If there's someone surrendering a #2 in the common work restroom—GIVE THEM SPACE. Put yourself in their shoes (poos—ugh, I hate myself for this stupid reference).

5. Don't eat someone else's food. I've never been a cook. I've never made myself food and then packed it up and kept it for future meals or brought it to work the next day. Instead, I've definitely gotten drunk and eaten my hyper-organized college roommate's food. It did not end well. People who make themselves pre-meals will be pissed when you eat their perfectly packed chicken Caesar salad wrap on a Friday afternoon. That person chose to work outside of work and make food—don't ruin that for them.

6. Be ambitious. Don't be afraid to speak up at meetings and/or offer your opinion(s) on projects. Apparently, drive is a quality bosses like in employees. Supposedly. *Drive* is also a pretty bad movie.

7. Dress appropriately for your work environment. We get it; you want everyone to know how creative and interesting you are. Well, let your personality do that for you rather than your crop top and feather shoes.

8. At the beginning, there's a lot of grunt work. It's likely that you'll be doing a lot of menial tasks when you start your professional career. Getting coffee, making copies, organizing closets, things a monkey with slightly above-average intelligence could do. Don't let it get to you. Get the coffee as best you can and persevere.

9. Keep your computer clean. I'm always hyper-paranoid about what people can and can't see on my computer screen. Or, when I was working on a company computer, what they could tap into and see in my search history. Don't set yourself up for an awkward situation—keep it clean.

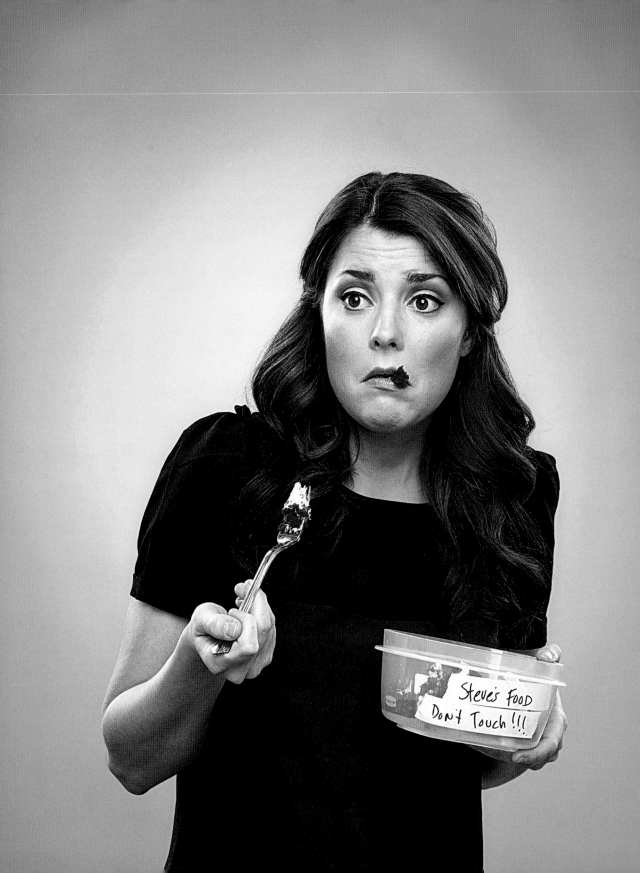

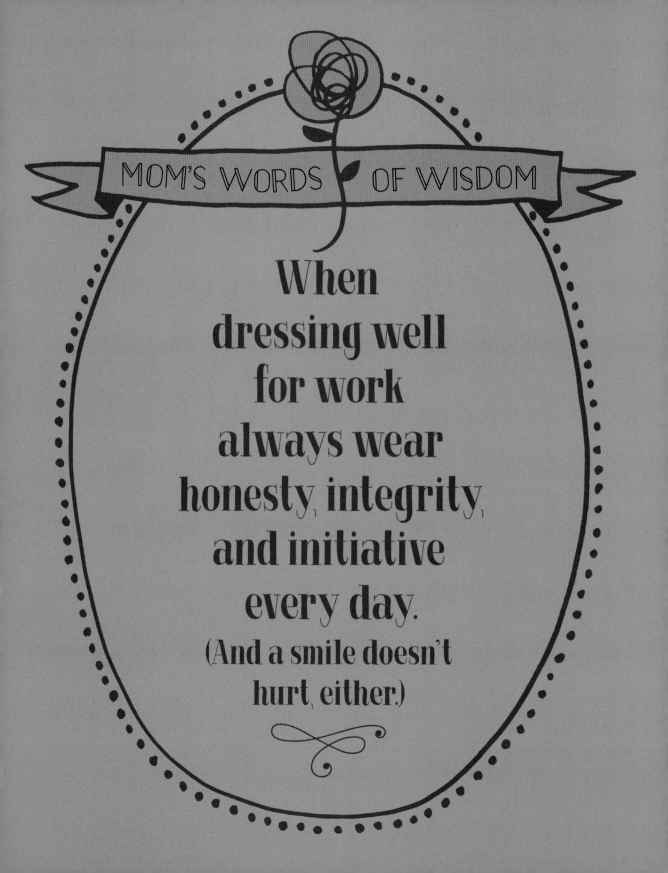

MOM'S WORDS OF WISDOM

When dressing well for work always wear honesty, integrity, and initiative every day. (And a smile doesn't hurt, either.)

10. Create an organization system. Figure out what works best for you to stay prepared and on-task. The person who created highlighters didn't do it for farts and giggles.

11. Ask for help if you need it. This was something I struggled with. I always wanted to prove I could handle things on my own and assumed that asking for help was some sort of sign of incompetence. Turns out, it isn't. Smart people ask for help, because it's a much more efficient way of doing things than wasting time doing it the wrong way.

12. Always be nice to the office weirdos. I mean, be nice to everyone all the time, but especially them. We're all just trying to get through this sh*t storm called life together. Remember that.

13. Be on time. I'm really terrible at this. But try. When you're late it can come across as you thinking your time is more important than someone else's. Don't give yourself an opportunity to give a wrong impression.

14. Use the office printer to your advantage, within reason. Buying ink when your home printer runs out is annoying; remember you can print things at work! Yay!

15. Office coffee is always pretty terrible. Unless you work at a coffee shop. I suggest outsourcing your caffeine intake.

16. Try to keep personal drama outside of your work world. It'll help you and your coworkers maintain sanity in the workplace. Plus, how annoyed do you get every time you hear Janice talk about her cat's emphysema? Right? Don't be that person.

17. Collaborate. Learn to work with others. It's something you'll have to do at some point in your professional career, so be an open and willing participant. Give and take, like a healthy digestive system. And pick up the phone every now and then. Email can be a time-suck and you often learn more/resolve issues faster on the phone—or even better, face-to-face.

18. Don't steal ideas; you're better than that.

19. Take criticism. Even if you don't agree with what someone says, be the bigger person.

20. Oh hey, if you don't like your job, you can quit! Imagine that! Maybe do it in some elaborate, comedic way and film it, and SLAM, you have a viral video. Now your new profession is: YouTuber. Congrats.

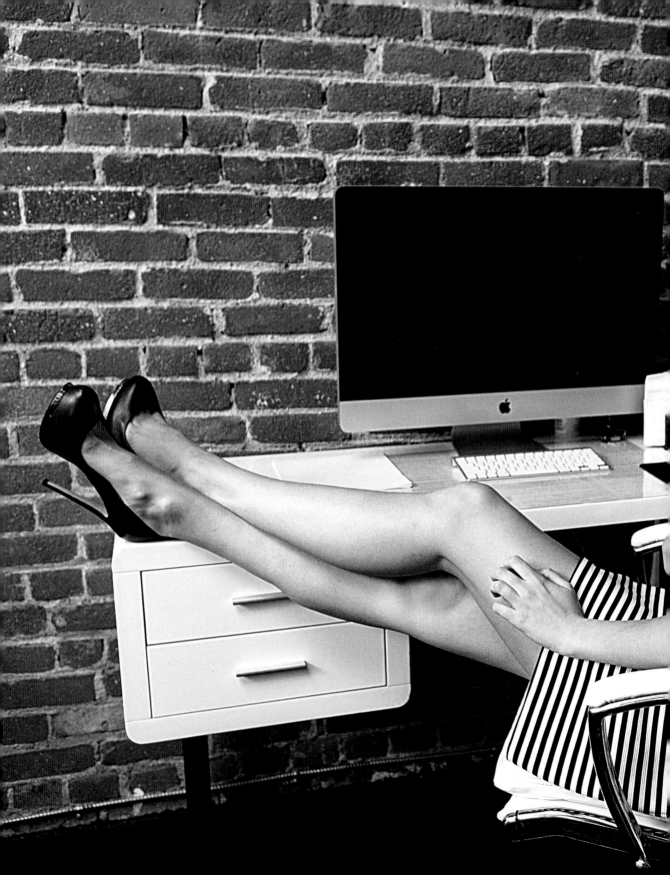

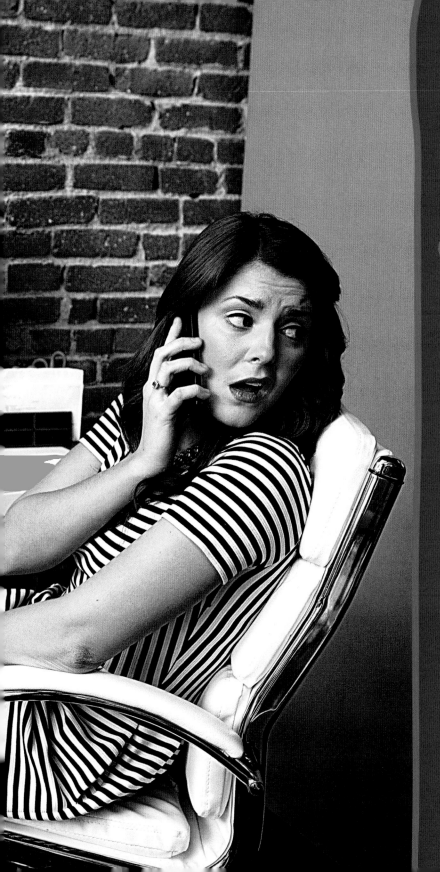

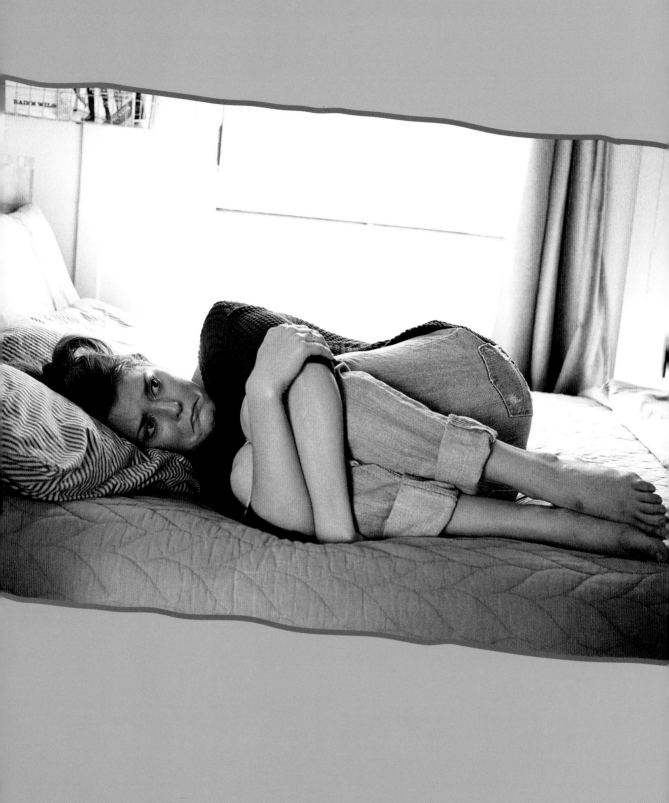

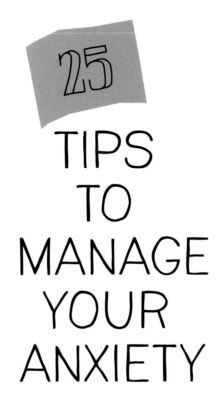

25 TIPS TO MANAGE YOUR ANXIETY

Over the last seven or eight years, I've been figuring out how to deal with my anxiety issues. Believe it or not, I'm a tremendously anxious person. Sometimes I think my entire body is one big nervous system, but my brother who studies science at MIT assures me that it's not. I'm still not convinced, Tim. Still not convinced.

I had anxiety issues before I even understood what anxiety was. When I was in high school, I was so shy. I think you could ask my entire graduating class if I ever spoke a word in the four years we spent together and 95 percent of them would say, "Wait, which girl are you asking me about?" or "Answer my question first, does Four Loko still have the booze in it or not?" (I'm from South Jersey.)

I thought college was going to be an opportunity to reinvent myself and become outgoing and interesting and FUN. But right from the start, I had trouble changing my hermit tendencies. I only hung out with my boyfriend at the time or occasionally with other people in super-small groups. I filled up my time with school and jobs to distract myself from the question: Should I try to hang out with someone? The thought of even putting myself out there to ask someone to hang out only to probably be rejected (I always assumed the worst-case scenario) was AWFUL. So instead, I always had something else to do. Even if I did go out, I'd leave when I felt overwhelmed and say that I had work in the morning or some project to finish.

After I graduated, I pursued my interest in improv and started coming out of my shell. Somehow pretending I was a horny monkey astronaut in front of an audience of a hundred-plus people helped. Not only did I start to feel like part of the comedy scene community, I was also going out to bars more regularly and doing something called "socializing." WHAT A CONCEPT. When I didn't want to hang out or had pangs of social anxiety, I'd stay home, make videos, and put them up on something called "YouTube." It was a way for me to express myself creatively and "perform" for an audience from the comfort of my own home. With or without pants. I only film myself from the waist up, you pervs.

For a few years things were pretty okay, but in 2010 I started getting those intense pangs again. In NYC, you're CONSTANTLY surrounded by people. All day. From morning 'til night. Even if you're going home at four a.m., there are people on the street. It's what makes the city so cool and what makes it so terrible, and the constant exposure to humans both sane and not so sane started affecting me.

I felt claustrophobic whenever I went outside. I even posted a video in 2010 on YouTube discussing my social anxiety, but in more of a joking way because I still didn't totally recognize what my feelings were. I thought I was just prone to nervousness and eventually my totally irrational, paralyzing fears would melt away.

NEGATRON.

It wasn't until about 2011 or 2012 that I really began to understand what was happening to me. I was dating a guy who had been diagnosed with an anxiety disorder when he was in college. With professional help, he discovered that the reason he had to walk out of parties to throw up in the front yard (sober) was because he was having panic attacks. Oh, there's an actual name for that feeling when you think you're having an early-onset heart attack and all the heat in your body rushes to your face! Oh duh! A panic attack.

He told me that he still got them from time to time, but learned breathing exercises to work through them. I felt relieved to know that I wasn't crazy. There was a name for the symptoms I was experiencing. And it was comforting to know I wasn't alone. Phew! These feelings are sure to melt away now!

NEGATRON.

For some reason as soon as I recognized that these moments weren't just onetime fleeting sensations, they started to occur more frequently. Just the anticipation of having a panic attack would trigger a panic attack. ACK. It was terrible. It got to the point that every time I got on the subway, I'd immediately sweat and my heart would pound in my ears. I'd feel so hot and claustrophobic that I'd have to jump out before I even got to my stop. The cool thing about New York is that even though I was sweating and turning red, I still wasn't the craziest-looking person on the train! Yay, diversity!

Then I started missing improv shows, because I just couldn't get myself to the theater. I was increasingly agitated by the unavoidable crowds every time I went out. The most frustrating part about my anxiety was the constant, obsessive, spiraling thoughts: *This didn't used to happen, just go back to being that other person who didn't overanalyze her anxious thoughts.* And I couldn't.

The saving grace of the situation (because, trust me, this Grace needed saving) was that I was

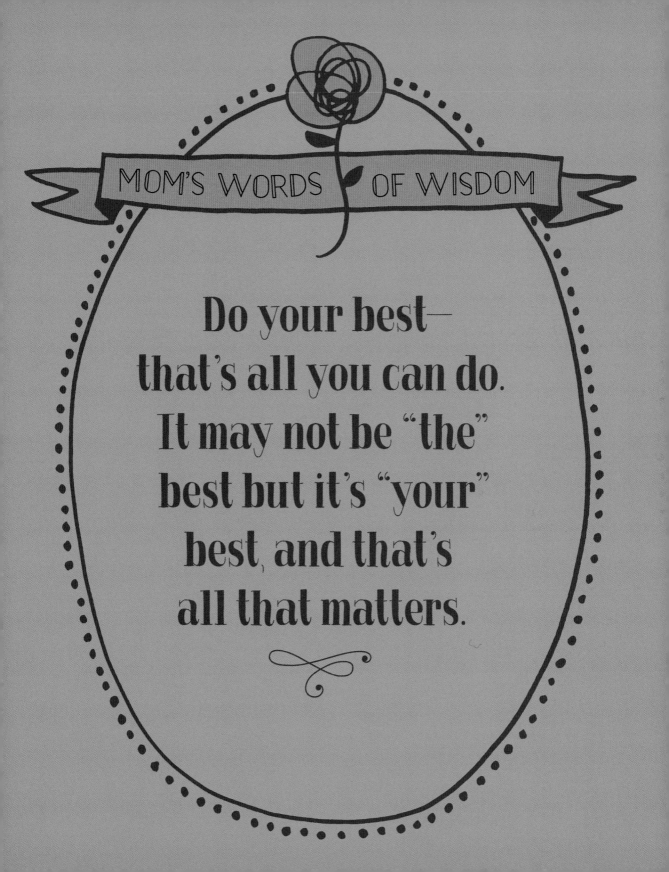

MOM'S WORDS OF WISDOM

Do your best—
that's all you can do.
It may not be "the"
best but it's "your"
best, and that's
all that matters.

planning to move to Los Angeles. I was getting out of this Escher-painting-of-anxiety hell soon!

My anxiety was still intense when I finally moved to Los Angeles, so I decided to get professional help. (I had tried a bunch of therapy in the past, but I was stupid about it. I would straight-up lie to my therapist and say, "Yeah, I did that thing you said and now I'm fine"—what an idiot.) I started seeing a psychiatrist and got prescribed some antidepressants and anti-anxiety medicine. They've really worked wonders for me. They're not for everyone, and I avoided seeing a psychiatrist for a long time, because I was nervous (when am I not?) about going the medication route. But, for me, it's made all the difference, along with some other (seemingly dumb but kind of effective) tips I've come up with on my own time.

DISCLAIMER: I'm not a doctor, nor do I play one on TV. These are just some suggested tips that have worked for me. If you're struggling with anxiety or other mental health issues, get professional help.

Here are twenty-five tips for managing your anxiety (it was going to be fifty, but I thought that might make you anxious):

1. **See a doctor.** If you're struggling, get help. Take your time to find someone that you feel comfortable with. This took me a second. It's like getting into a good relationship. A good relationship is one that makes you a better person. Also therapy can be stupid expensive, so, like a good lady of the night, get your money's worth.

2. **Remove yourself from a stressful situation.** When you're feeling anxious, don't be afraid to leave for a short period of time or completely. Sometimes, when I feel nervous on planes and the thought of the person next to me picking up on my nervous energy causes more nerves, I go to the bathroom to be alone and splash cold water on my face. Sure, now everyone waiting for the bathroom probably thinks you're taking a major-league dump, but hey, this is about you, not poo.

3. **BREATHE.** This is a "no doy!" tip, but sometimes I forget. When I check in with my body, I realize I've been breathing like an asthmatic that just ran a block. I try to make a conscious effort to focus my attention on deeper breathing. Like a poser type of meditation.

4. **Think about someone getting hit in the face with bread.** There's something about that visual that really takes my mind off

my anxiety. Maybe it's because my imagination has to work hard to figure out what possible scenario could actually make this happen IRL, or it's knowing that you can't really get hurt with bread, or it's because thinking of the different types of bread that would work best (loaf, pitas, English muffin, a single slice) is incredibly distracting. It's a great time if you really let yourself Wonder Bread. Sorry.

5. Exercise. Getting blood pumping through my body is a great stress reliever. Even if it's just jogging for ten minutes. My brain starts focusing on thoughts like, *Am I swallowing my own blood?* rather than, *I can't go to that party because I'll have a panic attack and all the cool people will see and I can never . . . oh god, here come the hives.*

6. Imagine someone walking by you with a cake and smashing that cake to the ground for no reason. This is one of my go-tos.

7. YouTube-search "people falling down slowly" or "men falling off boats." It will definitely divert your attention and give you some fun visuals to recall later if you start to feel nervous.

8. Scream and/or laugh and/or weep into a pillow. This is best to do privately.

9. Allow one person who makes you feel

completely comfortable to see you panic. Maybe this will help you start to find even the smallest ounce of comfort in your discomfort.

10. LOOK AT PUPPIES. In real life or on the Internet. If you can't find a puppy to be around in real life, I highly, HIGHLY recommend YouTube-searching "Sophie Rolls Down a Hill." It's my morning go-to pump-up video. She's truly an inspiration.

11. Rip up paper. Maybe only, like, one piece, so environmentalists don't get too anxious.

12. DANCE IT OUT. Put on your favorite jam and pump up the volume (god, I sound like a mom). I gravitate toward the song "Shake It Out" by Florence and the Machine, because it makes me feel mighty and powerful.

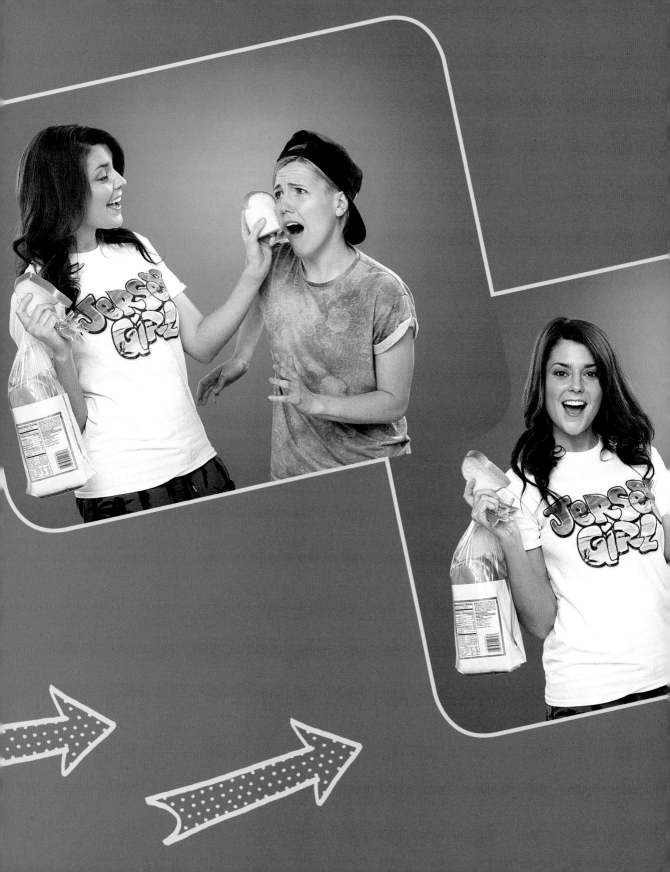

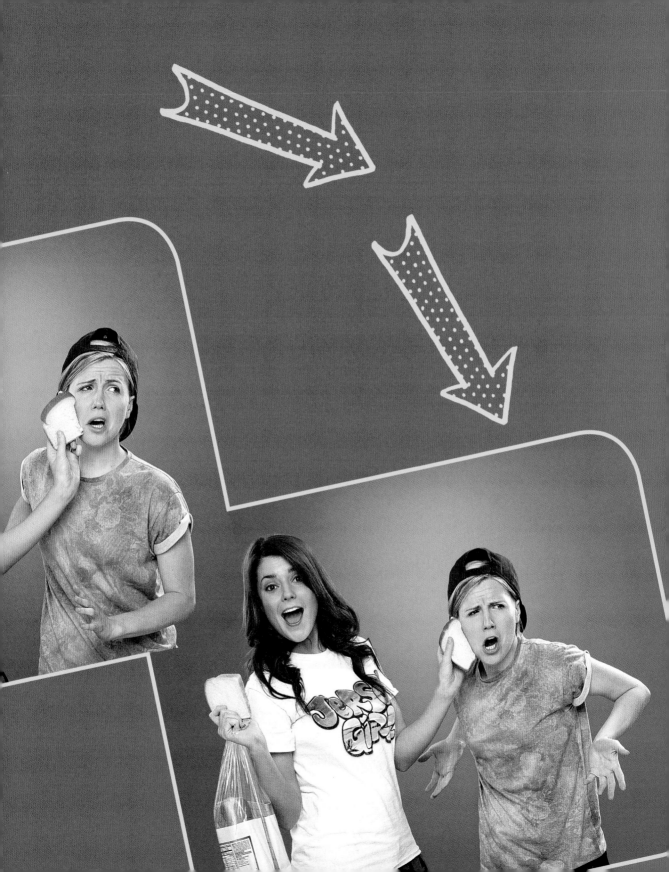

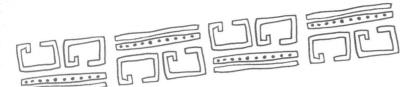

13. **Throw balled-up socks at the wall.**
It's therapeutic and socks can't really do too much damage to anything. Sometimes I imagine the socks are actually bouncing off Mario Batali's belly. It's a great use of a Sunday afternoon.

14. **Meditate.** HAHAHAHAHAHAHA, just kidding. Run into a meditation class and scream, "Meditate more like mediTAINT!" See what happens.

15. **Lie on the floor and stare at your ceiling.** Let your brain drift off into thought. Maybe imagine a world where *Supermarket Sweep* still exists. Maybe imagine grabbing a cold beer with that chill dog from *The Never-Ending Story*.

16. **This is for all of you *The Price Is Right* lovers.** Find a quiet place (or even add this on to #15) where you can imagine the Plinko chip falling gently into the $10,000 slot over and over and over again. And then visualize a slightly overweight, middle-aged woman with white sneakers, spandex leggings, and a puffy painted shirt that says DREW CAREY ME AWAY TO THE SHOW-CASE SHOWDOWN! flashing the audience.

17. **Pee in the shower listening to "Let It Go."**

18. **Write a letter to your anxious self.** Describe what it's like on the other side of panic. Panic attacks can last minutes or they can last hours, and the relief that comes on the other side is so sweet. But when you're in the middle of an attack, it's almost impossible to recall that calm state. So, try to write it down to the best of your ability and see what you come up with. Maybe even mail it to yourself if you're that kind of freak.

19. **Watch cooking shows on mute listening to Celine Dion.** Food has never looked so emotional.

20. **Wrap yourself up in a blanket and roll around on the floor like a human taco.** I love this. It makes me feel like a dumb child and I don't care, it's so much fun to let yourself go.

BONUS: For those experiencing a panic attack, here are some

EMERGENCY BRIEF RELIEFS

▫ REMEMBER: UNLIKE THAT MOVIE *CASINO ROYALE*, IT WON'T LAST FOREVER.

▫ HOW DO YOU THINK A CAVE-MAN REACTED THE FIRST TIME HE GOT A BONER?

▫ WHATEVER TERRIBLENESS YOU'RE EXPERIENCING RIGHT NOW, THERE'S PRESUMABLY SOMEONE ELSE IN THE WORLD WHO HAS EXPLOSIVE DIARRHEA AND IS LOCKED OUT OF HER HOUSE—YOU'RE WINNING.

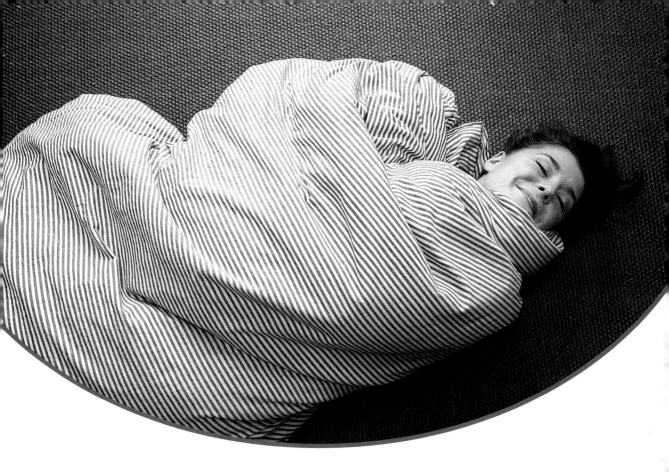

21. Throw large rocks into water and imagine it's the sound of giants taking dumps. It'll be so stupid and gross that you'll forget you're anxious. Also maybe do this with friends, so the other well-adjusted people at the park don't think you're a threat.

22. Make up a song about yourself. It doesn't matter if you have no musical aptitude— the worse the better. BUT the chorus has to be, "I'm a stinky turd/yeah you heard/I'm a stinky turd/oh yeah yeah turd is the word." Best of luck to you! And you're welcome in advance for landing that record deal.

23. CRAFT! Get your brain and hands focused on a project.

24. Plunge your hands into a barrel of coffee beans. Or a bowl of dried rice or a can of marbles. Yes, I know you think I'm insane, but IT FEELS VERY NICE AND SOOTHING SOMEHOW. I wouldn't say you should go to Whole Foods and compromise all the coffee bean barrels with your extremities, but buy some to take home and have fun.

25. Reread this book. Peh heh heh.

THE ART OF AVOIDING A
PUBLIC PANIC ATTACK

THE ART OF MAKING ADULT FRIENDS
AND INFLUENCING THEM
(TO REMAIN YOUR FRIEND)

THE ART OF BEING AROUND OTHER PEOPLE
FOR MORE THAN A FEW MINUTES

THE ART OF TRICKING YOURSELF
INTO ENJOYING TIME WITH OTHERS

THE ART OF FORCING YOURSELF OFF OF TUMBLR

The Art of Talking to Other Humans

~~THE ART OF EXISTING IN A PLACE THAT ISN'T YOUR HOME/BED/COMPUTER CHAIR~~

~~THE ART OF STEPPING OUT YOUR FRONT DOOR AND THEN TAKING A FEW MORE STEPS~~

Your Social Life

Here's where I'll try to teach you about cool, hip, young, fun stuff.

Welcome to the social section. Here's where I'll try to teach you about cool, hip, young, fun stuff like throwing a party and making adult friends and hanging out by yourself. Because these are all things I have in fact done! Woo! I've reached some level of personal/social development! It's been a long time coming. I used to be very low-functioning in terms of socializing.

My sophomore year of college, my long-term boyfriend broke up with me and I sloppy-cried for a week. And then I decided to do something for myself. I had always wanted to go overseas, so I signed up for a study abroad in London for three and a half weeks over the winter break. I was going by myself, which was a huge deal for me. At the initial orientation, I sort of knew another girl who had also registered by herself, so we decided to room together. She was pretty nerdy and quiet like me. *Wait, was I making a friend?*

I was nineteen at the time and the legal drinking age in London is eighteen. Uh-oh. We were required to take one class for three college credits. The class was from ten a.m. until one p.m. every day in the same building as the dorms. After the class, we were free to do whatever we wanted. There was also a pub on campus whose **happy hour started at four-thirty every day. Double uh-oh.**

The first night, the program leader (aka the dorm's American RA, who thought he was cooler than he actually was and was very openly trying to sleep with any and all of the girls in the program)

organized a trip for all of us to go to a dance club. It was so stupid. He told us that it was free drinks all night and dancing. The reality was that it was one free drink with sweaty thirty-year-old men grinding on your back. My response to the situation was to get drunk and accidentally break two glasses.

That night, I met a guy who was a production assistant at MTV. At that time, I thought that was *so* cool. Now that I've actually done a few internships at MTV transcribing interviews for *My Super Sweet 16*, I realize that it was *not* an impressive pick-up line.

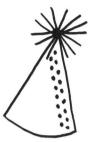

The next night, my roommate and I decided to break off from the RA's planned evening activity and venture down to the campus pub. We found another couple we both "sort of" knew already drinking (that's the thing about going to a small school—everyone "sort of" knows each other). They were cool and funny and very hipster-y. I liked them and I really wanted them to like me. We all got super drunk with the on-campus bartender and it was great. I remember thinking the bartender was cute right away. At the end of the night, I introduced him to MySpace and showed him my profile and I was so proud—what a nerd.

We continued the getting-drunk-with-the-campus-bartender routine the next couple of nights until we eventually ventured farther out beyond campus to a bar in an area called Camden Town that the couple heard was cool. It was bartended by five attractive Australians who all lived together in the apartment upstairs. It was an Australian, male Coyote Ugly in London. Triple uh-oh! It was also kind of an indie rock/hipster bar full of guys and girls in bands with tattoos and faded leather jackets and ALL THE CIGARETTES. I stood out like a pig on a plane.

The bartenders and regulars nicknamed me the Cheerleader, because I dressed in bright-colored clothing from the Gap and got really happy when I was drunk. I'd never felt cooler. I quickly developed a crush on a scrawny, sweet British bar regular named Tom. I was a repressed single girl abroad; this was THE BEST.

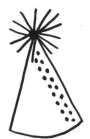

The rest of the trip was a wonderful blur of getting drunk in the school's pub with my campus bartender crush and then going out in Camden Town to my new favorite Aussie hole-in-the-wall to be around my other indie infatuation. Some highlights included getting so drunk in the campus pub that I spent the night walking up and down my dorm hallway spitting on the carpet and cursing out the bartender to no one. I sobered up when I spat right next to a girl I hadn't seen walking down the hallway and she said, "Ew, are you okay?" I said, "YES, I'M FINE, ARE YOU OKAY?"

Another night I saw a stray dog pass the Australian bar and I followed it outside and around the block for a half hour before indie bar regular Tom came and collected me. He wouldn't let me keep the dog. That was his only flaw. Another night, a too-cool rocker regular named Ollie tried to argue with me about "what an idiot George Bush is." I was never someone who talked about politics (I know my limitations), so I did a cartwheel away from this conversation and he laughed and bought me a shot. I felt like I was really taking on the role of the Cheerleader, like it was some sort of superhero alter ego. I felt free and fun.

The last night of the trip, the fun couple, my roommate, and I went out and somehow my roommate got separated from us. A bartender told us she left with a guy she had been talking to for the past couple nights. *Get it quiet, nerdy roommate!* Tom couldn't come out that night, because he had a business thing (the memory is blurry), so the fun couple and I met up with the campus bartender and ended up drinking back at his place.

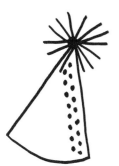

I fell asleep on the couch with him (there was no sex because I was still shy and sheltered, but at the end of the day I still felt scandalous, and that was enough for me). He took me back to campus in the morning, I kissed him good-bye, and had to pack up my stuff to leave right away. Once I took a second to look around the room in my hungover stupor, I realized my roommate still wasn't back. Uh-oh. We were all waiting in the lobby ready to go to the airport when she finally walked through the front door with messy hair, avoiding all eye contact. She grabbed all of her stuff as quickly as she could and met us back in the lobby. I whispered, "Are you okay?" and she replied, "It was awesome."

As we flew back that day, I remember feeling different. Part of the feeling was because I was wildly hungover. But I was also feeling pride, because I'd expanded my horizons and allowed myself to experience fun times with new people. It was the first moment in my adult life that I thought, *Oh, I can do this whole "social" thing.* And I've tried to keep it going ever since. There've been peaks and valleys and mountains and beaches and canyons and strip malls, but here are some of the things I've picked up along the way. And none of them are STDs!

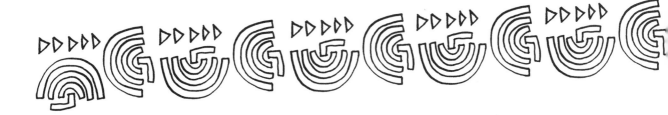

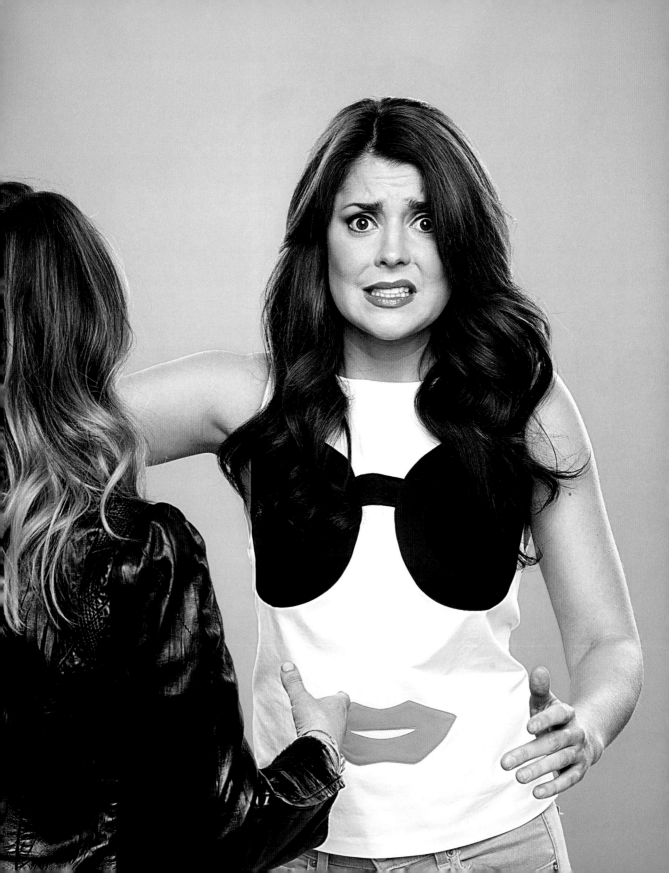

HOW TO
MAKE ADULT FRIENDS

Ever since I can remember, I've had this irrational notion that there's only a short window of time to make friends and then I'd just sort of . . . have them for the rest of my life. I never thought that I could make new friends as an adult. I'd be way too busy doing my taxes or picking out the classiest briefcase. I could have acquaintances or people I saw occasionally and whose company I enjoyed, but making new friends as a grownup just didn't happen. Welcome to my stunted socialization.

I've never been great at making friends. (Does this sound like a sob story, or do I just sound self-aware?) Putting myself out there was never my strong suit (I prefer a blazer and jeans—LOL). My parents have been divorced since I was a tiny, one-eighth-formed human. Every other weekend I was at my dad's house away from my friends, so I missed a lot of hangout opportunities. Which was fiiiiiine by me—I preferred to

spend time with my family rather than enter the social gauntlet. However, by the time I reached eleventh or twelfth grade, my social circles were more like social dots. I could count my friends on one hand (if that), which was still okay by me. I've never been the person with a hundred friends. Maintaining that many relationships makes me anxious (but what doesn't?).

When I got to college, reality smacked me in the butt with a wet towel. Reality is kinda pervy. I was on my own and forced to try to make new friends—except I had ABSOLUTELY NO IDEA how to do it. I hung out with very few people in high school, and we were all on the same end of the underdeveloped socialization spectrum. In college, I remember sort of trying to hang out and talk to the people on my floor, but ultimately I was too shy and nervous to see any of those relationships through. I used to sit on my bed at night and actually try to break down the act of making a friend. Does it happen when you find a common interest? Or when you're introduced by someone else? Or does it require witchcraft? I felt like a socially undeveloped loser. Why didn't they teach a class freshman year called "Here Are Some Friends, Now Go Be Less Sad"?

I just wanted someone to give me a guidebook. I spent weeks going to the student center, looking at the corkboard with flyers to sign up for student-run clubs, thinking, *Friends could happen because of clubs, right?* I signed up for a couple and it turns out I don't really enjoy volunteering or peer mediation. At least I learned that about myself.

Eventually I started making friends with like-minded comedy folk—extremely slowly and sort-of-but-not-really steadily. And by the end of college I felt like I had some friends, but I still had no idea how it had happened.

After college, I moved to Brooklyn and got into the improv scene. The comedy community really helped me, but *you-can't-make-friends-as-an-adult* still flashed through my mind. I was cordial with everyone, but apprehensive about hanging out with the people I met at the comedy club. That changed when I met Mamrie Hart.

Mamrie was on my first-ever sketch comedy team in 2007. We performed together for a few months and were friendly but never really got together outside of meetings, rehearsals, or shows. One weekday afternoon after the team disbanded for the day, Mamrie asked me if I wanted to get a Bloody Mary in the Brooklyn neighborhood that we both lived in. We didn't have day jobs (modern women). My usual nervous self was super anxious—Mamrie

was confident and funny and a bartender—she was too cool for me. But I agreed and it was great! And then we hung out again, and another time, and voilà, we were friends! Now we work together on a ton of projects and we've even had diarrhea while sharing a hotel room. FRIENDS!

Over the past few years most of my closest friends have come from the people I've met as an "adult." The following aren't rules to live by, because friends are made in spontaneous ways. These are just loose guidelines for finding friendship as a grown-up.

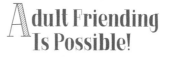

Adult Friending Is Possible!

Recognize this fact: it's possible to make friends as an adult.

Maybe you know this already, and maybe I'm the only baby-lady that still has to convince herself that this is true. It is true. At this point in your life you've had experiences, you have opinions, and therefore you're ripe to find meaningful new relationships with positive people who will enrich your life. This is the best time to make friends! They get to know your true self instead of your awkward, going-through-puberty self. You can legally drink together! You can grow old and cranky together.

Put Out

Not sexually.

That is not a way to make friends. That is a way to make awkwards. And it's not fun to hang out with awkwards more than once. Put yourself out there and make yourself available for camaraderie. It took me a while to realize that "you only get what you give" is an insightful song lyric about companionship and not solely about Christmas presents. You can't win in a casino unless you place a bet. (Side note: Casinos aren't the worst place to make friends; house fires are probably the worst place.)

nitiate

Take a chance.
Initiate some sort of hangout. I'm awful at this. I'm so stupidly afraid of being the one to suggest something. But in tandem with the last step (and unlike me, and more like Doritos), be bold. You don't have to specify exactly what you want to do or where you want to go, but just letting the person know you want to spend time with them is part of the friend-making process. It helps to remind myself that maybe they feel the same way that I do and they're hoping I'll initiate a hang.

It's like when you have a litter of puppies and you're like, "Would anyone want one of these puppies?" and some random is like, "You know what, now that you've said something, I would love a puppy. Thank you." Boom. Best friends. You and the other person and the dog forever.

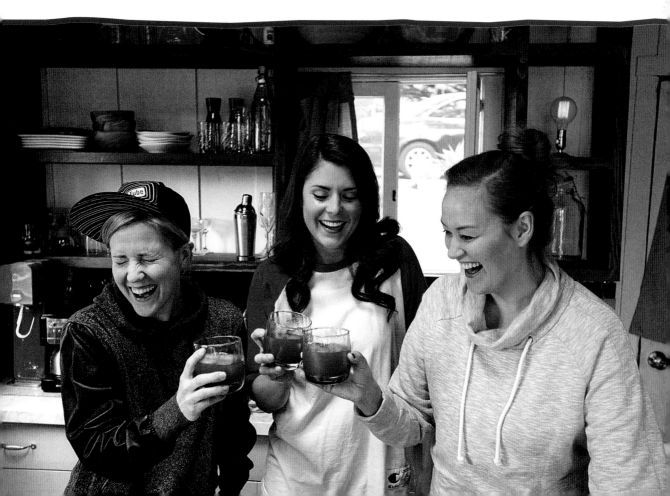

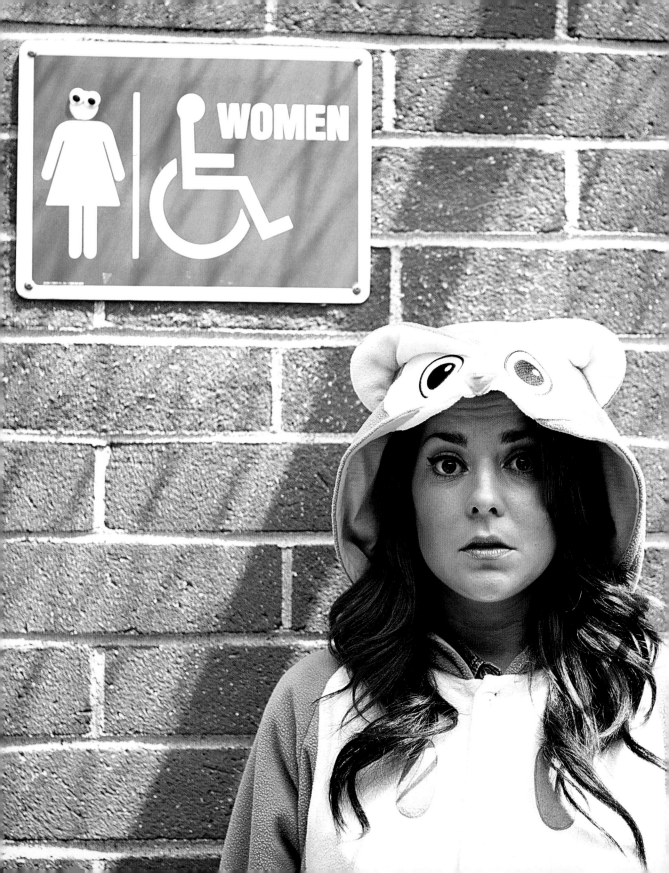

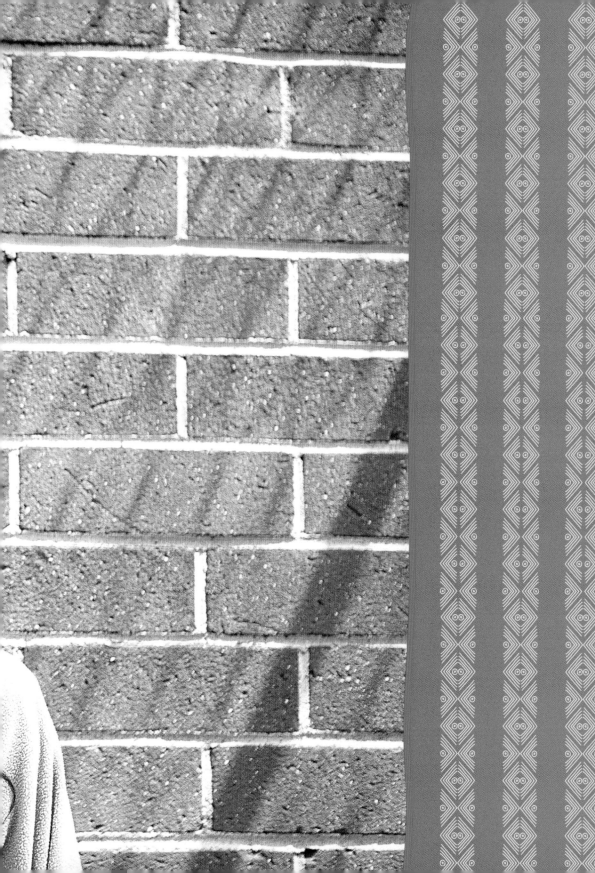

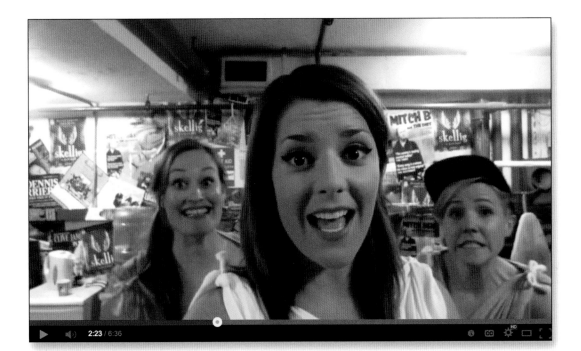

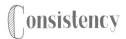

Common Interests

People who share your interests could equal future potential friends.

This seems like a "no doy" entrée with a side of "what else is new" sauce and some "omg, srsly?" for dessert. It's an incredibly basic principle, but some of the most basic ideas yield the greatest results (see: macaroni and cheese).

When I joined the improv community and again when I became part of the YouTube community, I met some of my best friends. Who knew that connecting over similar experiences or talking about a mutual hobby could lead to friendship? Why don't they teach this in kindergarten?

Like that person's shirt? Ask him about it. He might become your best man. Who knows? The universe is ridiculous.

Ketchup

We go together like . . .

Surround yourself with people who are the ketchup to your french fries—they make you a better version of yourself. Yes, french fries are amazing on their own, but combined with ketchup they're a force. Spend time with the people who bring out your true flavors but don't overpower you.

Consistency

Hang out consistently.

My two best friends and I have a stupid relationship—if we don't see each other once every three days we assume one of us drunkenly fell into a mall fountain. Being a cool friend with

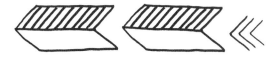

someone requires time and attention. Friends are like human dogs or human plants—pay them attention, buy them rawhides sometimes, and they'll love you forever(ish).

Open Yourself Up

Let's get deep.

Building a close friendship with someone is about opening yourself up to the other person and vice versa. Sharing a deeper part of yourself with another human being is a special experience. And when you have a certain level of trust and feel comfortable sharing your private information/thoughts with them, it only deepens the bond. It's a free, fun form of therapy! The greatest friends are the ones who want to listen and share. You're not truly friends until you've heard about the time they shat behind a school bus.

Pool

Everyone jump in!

Get everyone in the pool! Start mixing and matching friends and hangouts. It creates more opportunities to keep things interesting and meet other people. You never really know who you'll hit it off with, and if you put yourself out there into other "pools" of people you might meet someone cool. Every now and then, someone will take a piss in the pool—kick those people out. Otherwise, it's a party! Pools are cool.

Here are some inspirational **hangout ideas** you can do with your adult friends:

- Bloody Mary party: Create a Bloody Mary bar and let your friends make their own. This way people can make alcoholic and nonalcoholic beverages alike. Also maybe have other options for drinks because Bloody Marys can be very polarizing.
- Theme parks and/or laser tag: Even when you're an adult this is a really fun time. Also, it's an educational experience. At the last theme park I went to, I found out my body can only handle so many roller coasters before my neck and lower back inform me that they are in fact older and crumblier than they were in high school.
- Board game night: People like games because they don't require any physical activity—they're the great equalizer!
- Themed dinner party: Why just eat food when you could eat food dressed as a NYC tourist or in German lederhosen? When people watch sports in jerseys, they're basically doing athletic cosplay, so why not make your dinner parties just as fun and stupid?
- Hiking/river rafting/camping/general outdoor stuff: Some people like being outside. Neat and ew.

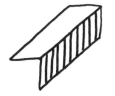

Remember:

A PICK(Y) COP

Adult Friending Is Possible!

Put Out
Initiate
Common Interests
Ketchup

Consistency
Open Yourself Up
Pool

#APICKYCOP

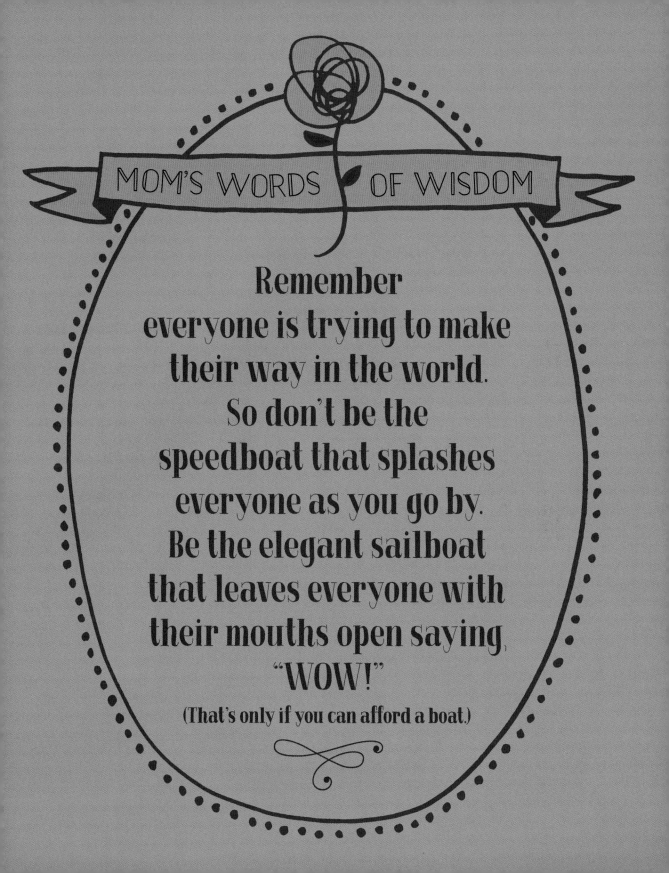

MOM'S WORDS OF WISDOM

Remember
everyone is trying to make
their way in the world.
So don't be the
speedboat that splashes
everyone as you go by.
Be the elegant sailboat
that leaves everyone with
their mouths open saying,
"WOW!"

(That's only if you can afford a boat.)

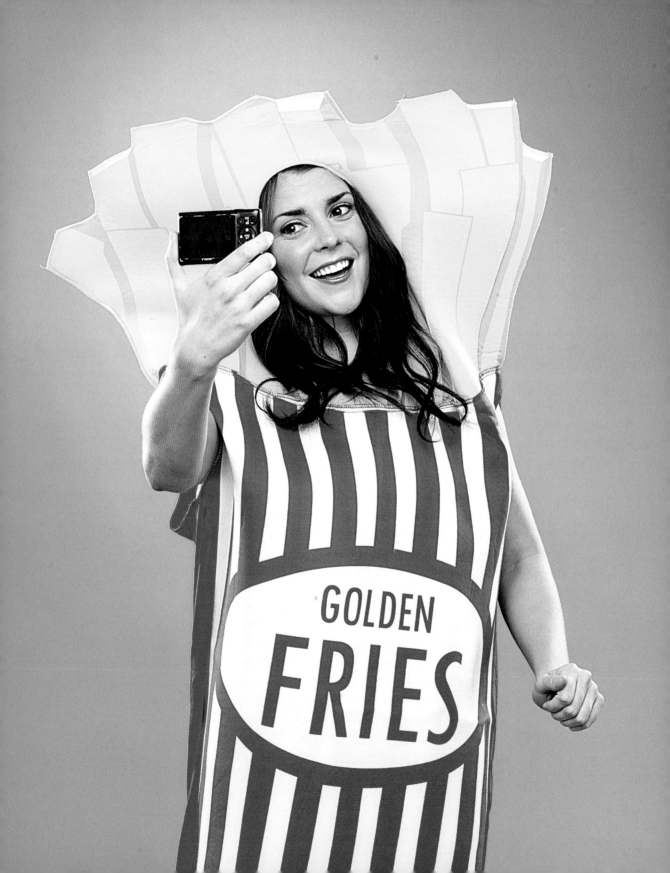

HOW TO
HANG OUT BY YOURSELF

Hanging out by myself is one of my all-time favorite activities and also one of my special skills—along with avoiding having to wear pants.

I'm a full-fledged introvert, which according to Urban Dictionary means: "A person who is energized by spending time alone. Often found in their homes, libraries, quiet parks that not many people know about, or other secluded places, introverts like to think and be alone."

All of that is true about me, except for the library part. Though I used to study in the basement floor of the library when I was in college, because I could fart/learn in solitude there.

It takes a lot of mental gymnastics to get me in the right headspace to go to a party or social event when I know I could have a GREAT time at home by myself with my dog and my solo dancing. At home, I can let it all hang out without judgments—although my dog gives AMAZING side eye, which keeps me in check. I love being alone, I prefer it nine times out of nine and a half. Attending parties and social events makes me incredibly anxious and afraid. It's probably why I got into vlogging—an inherently solitary activity. My vlogging started as a hobby; I used to hang out solo and record myself for fun. Now it's my full-time job. What a psychopath.

Hanging by myself might be the one thing in my life I've done the most, other than pooing, sleeping, or forgetting friends' and family members' birthdays. I'm a real treat. This is probably the only subject in the book that I'd actually consider myself to be an expert on.

You might think there's no technique to hanging out alone, but without preparation it can easily go from a fun time to a sobbing self-pity party. Those are the parties you never RSVP to, but by the end of the night you just sort of find yourself there. So do yourself a favor and consider this advice next time you want to paint your town(home) red.

Accept

Accept that this is what you're doing tonight.

It's a you, yourself, and also you festivity! This is going to be fun. You should be positive about this. Even if you're the most social human on the planet (I'm looking at you, Tyler Oakley), it's nice to retreat and recharge. Once you've made the decision to do so, you can release whatever social stress you might be carrying about having to go out or needing to see other living, breathing humans.

This is the whole reason the Internet exists— so you can catch up with someone by silently stalking their social media rather than talking to them in the real world! There will be other times for you to see them in the flesh. Just don't die tonight is all. Go you!

The only person you're responsible for pleasing tonight is yourself. And you know exactly what it takes to please you. Hopefully. Unless you're extremely self-hating, then maybe you shouldn't hang out by yourself. Probably better for you to be around others. Please skip to the next chapter. Everyone else, continue reading!

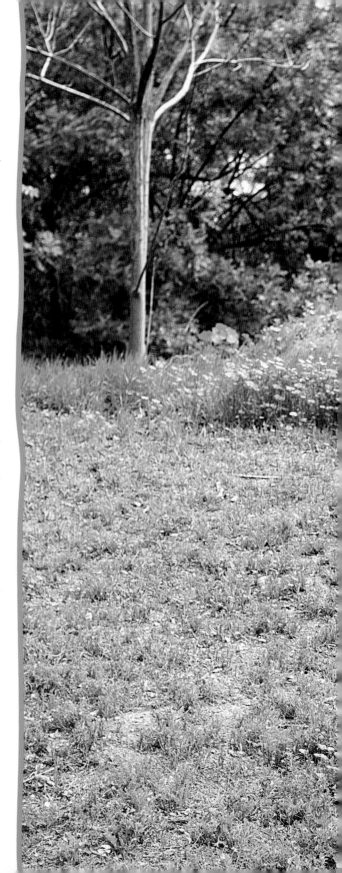

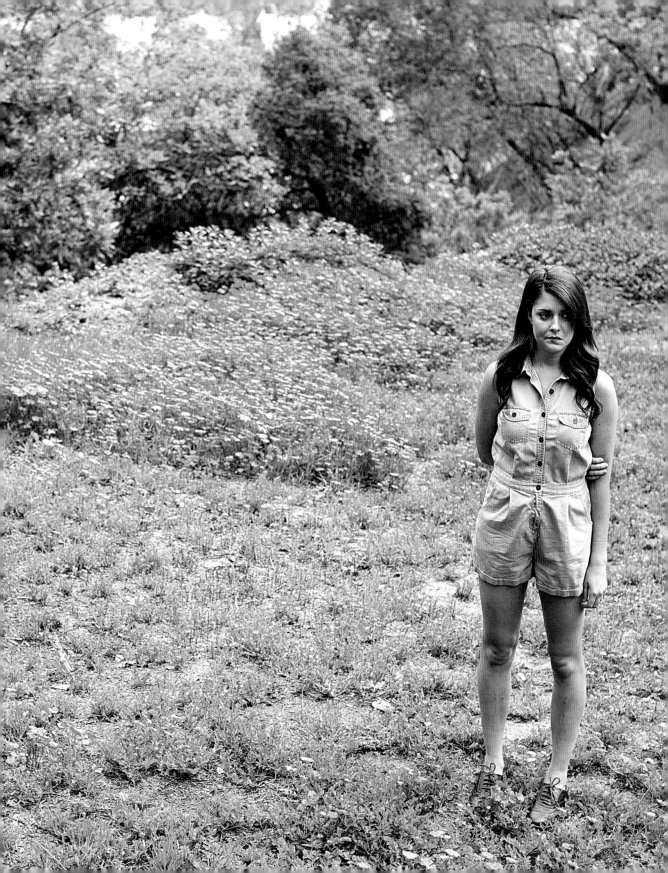

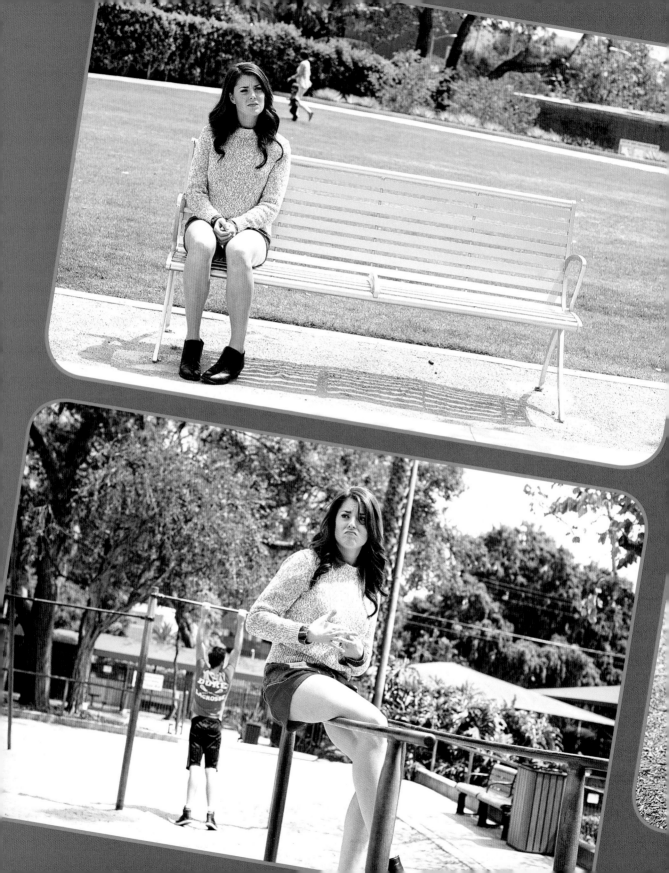

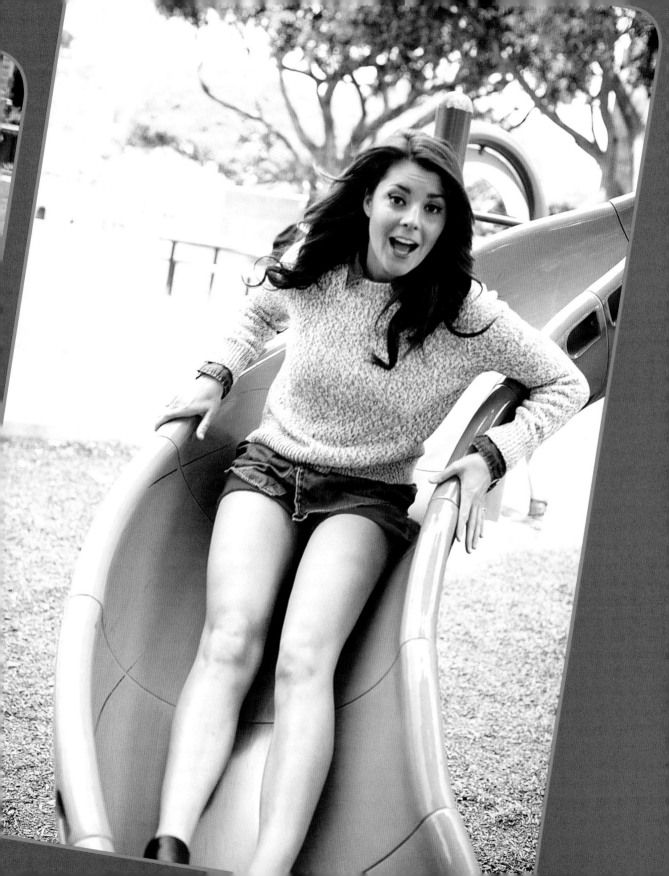

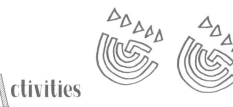

Stock up

Get supplies.

Stock up on the supplies you'll need and want tonight, so you don't have to leave your place at any point and "interact" with people. Here are some things that are helpful to have on hand:

○ Toilet paper—for sh*ts and giggles.
○ Food—for food.
○ WiFi—the French call it "wee-fee." True story.
○ Batteries—for the moment your mouse dies as you're Facebook-stalking "that girl" and you're just about to finally get to her not-so-flattering photos.
○ First-aid supplies—for oops.

Treat yourself to a movie-montage-style SHOPPING SPREE to get stuff to make your night magical.

Indulge

Tonight is YOUR night!

Ain't no party like a one-person party! I know that sounds omega dumb, but you can get away with saying things like that when you're alone. Treat yourself to the scandalous stuff you don't normally treat yourself to. Sweets, sweet weenies (self-serving YouTube video reference), sweats, Swift (Taylor), Swedish Fish, pornography . . . the list goes on.

When I'm alone, I usually allow/encourage myself to fall into K-holes of watching YouTube videos of French bulldog puppies mixed with beauty gurus in addition to watching any new episode of *The Real Housewives*. Some real highbrow stuff.

Activities

It's helpful to have activities to keep you occupied.

Also remember that when you're alone, there's no one to keep you from entering your mental Death Star. That bad mental space that locks you in and shoots lasers of depressing thoughts at you. Also, let it be known that I Googled "the deathstar is the bad one?" just for that last sentence. You're welcome, anyone who looks through my Google search history.

Plan some activities that will help you feel even the slightest bit productive and therefore satisfied about your night the next day. I lean toward basic things like laundry, washing dishes, exercising, writing the sequel to *It Takes Two* called *Actually, It Takes Three*, starring the Olsen twins and myself as triplets separated at birth who find each other as adults in NYC when they all apply to work at a bar called Coyote Average-Looking. None of us get the gig, but instead Ashley (whose character's name is Melissa Rivers) decides they should band together to score the biggest heist of their lives. Rob the bar. They call themselves River's 3. Everyone dies in the end, but in the opening scene Mary-Kate does meth off a homeless man's taint.

Slow

No need to rush anything tonight.

Take your time. Do absolutely nothing for hours if you want to. There isn't a right way to have a night to yourself. But there are some potential wrong ways, like: setting your house on fire, setting your neighbors' house on fire, trying to actually set fire to the rain, and so on and so forth.

Go at your own pace tonight. This is a marathon you're going to win no matter what. You don't have to worry about the girl or guy next to you with the made-for-running arm Spanx. What do those do? At first, I thought a lot of marathon runners were just embarrassed by their 2 percent of forearm fat.

I thrive on getting stuff done and overworking myself. The bags under my eyes wouldn't fit into an overhead luggage compartment (HEYO!). So on nights when I know I'm having "me" time, I try to remind myself that I don't HAVE to get that project done tonight. It will still be waiting for me in the morning.

Humor

Inject some ha-ha's into your night.

Watch something funny, do something funny, READ something funny. Scientists say that laughter burns calories and decreases your risk of all the cancers. By scientists I mean that last time I hung out by myself, I put on a lab coat and told myself that was a fact.

Accountable

You can't blame anyone else tonight.

So you need to be accountable for your actions and maybe create some personal ground rules—especially when it comes to expressing yourself via social media. I've had some solo-ragers that have ended with me tweeting complete and utter nonsense that in my head I thought was HILARIOUS. Here are just a couple of my favorites (please RT).

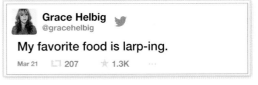

Grace Helbig
@gracehelbig

My favorite food is larp-ing.

Mar 21   207   1.3K   ...

I think my thought process was that larp sort of sounded like lard?

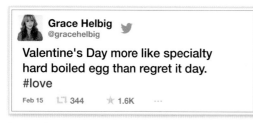

Grace Helbig @gracehelbig

Valentine's Day more like specialty hard boiled egg than regret it day. #love

Feb 15   344   1.6K

I guess I was upset that hard-boiled eggs have been making a comeback in restaurants, but why I associated them with Valentine's Day, I HAVE NO IDEA.

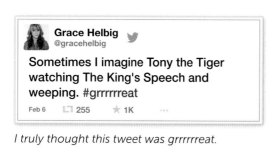

Grace Helbig @gracehelbig

Late night sincere twitter moment. (NO HACKS) @mametown & @harto are like THE BEST fondu. & your body doesn't have a lactose issue.

Feb 8   214   1.3K

I started my day hanging out and drinking with @harto and @mametown and then I went home for a solo night and let myself feel things.

Grace Helbig @gracehelbig

Sometimes I imagine Tony the Tiger watching The King's Speech and weeping. #grrrrrreat

Feb 6   255   1K

I truly thought this tweet was grrrrrreat.

Vicariousness

I don't know if this is a word, but it is now. This step is for all those who from time to time (myself included) like to torture themselves by deep-diving into someone else's (no doubt highly curated) social media profiles. I'm giving you the permission you need to go forth and prosper . . . I mean go forth and properly Internet-stalk. Whether it's someone you want to date or someone you want to hate or someone you want to bait (to be your best friend, because they are too awesome to be true), go nuts.

Investigate that Instagram, tap that Twitter, frisk that Facebook, and pass judgment on that Pinterest. BUT be safe. Don't "socially awkward penguin" yourself by accidentally typing the person's name into your status update, or unintentionally leaving a comment on that person's wall, or liking/RT-ing a post. Let yourself fall down the rabbit hole, but make sure you have a rope to climb out.

Emotional

Later in the evening, let the emotions fly. One of the greatest things about being alone is that you can let it all out. Whatever's bothering you, whatever's making you happy—feel it and enjoy the expression of emotion. This isn't necessarily for everyone. I'm a relatively reserved person in my normal life and I enjoy being alone so I can check my emotional temperature and see where I'm at without feeling uncomfortable.

My friends and I joke a lot about how when we're sad about something or just PMS-ing about nothing, we intensify all the feelings with the help of YouTube videos about surprise wedding proposals or soldiers reuniting with their dogs. Maybe we're crazy, but sometimes it's fun to cry. For me, I always feel a little lighter afterward. Do tears have calories?

Dance

This is the BEST part of the night. Dance like no one's watching. BECAUSE THEY AREN'T.

Remember:

ASIA SHAVED

Accept

Stock up

Indulge

Activities

Slow

Humor

Accountable

Vicariousness

Emotional

Dance

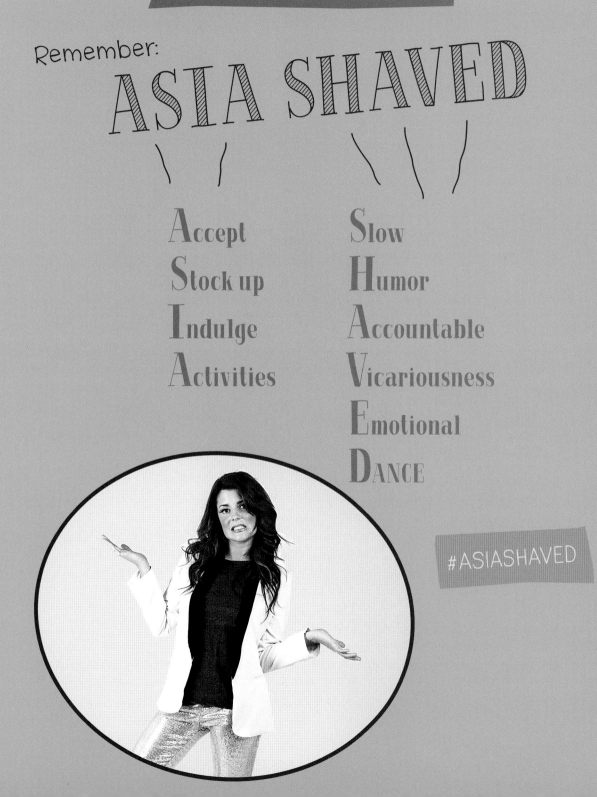

#ASIASHAVED

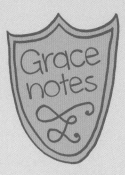
Grace notes

HOW TO HANG OUT BY YOURSELF

HOUR ONE CHECK-IN

1. Have you done anything productive? If so, what?
_____

2. What social media sites have you been on and what were you doing?
_____

3. How are you feeling emotionally and physically?
_____

HOUR TWO CHECK-IN

1. Have you done anything productive? If so, what?
_____

2. What social media sites have you been on and what were you doing?
_____

3. How are you feeling emotionally and physically?
_____

HOUR THREE CHECK-IN

1. Have you done anything productive? If so, what?
_____

2. What social media sites have you been on and what were you doing?
_____

3. How are you feeling emotionally?
_____

HOUR FOUR CHECK-IN

1. Get off social media. This is not a question, this is a command.
_____

2. Seriously, you've Internet-stalked that person enough. You're done.
_____

3. OMG SRSLY STOP.
_____

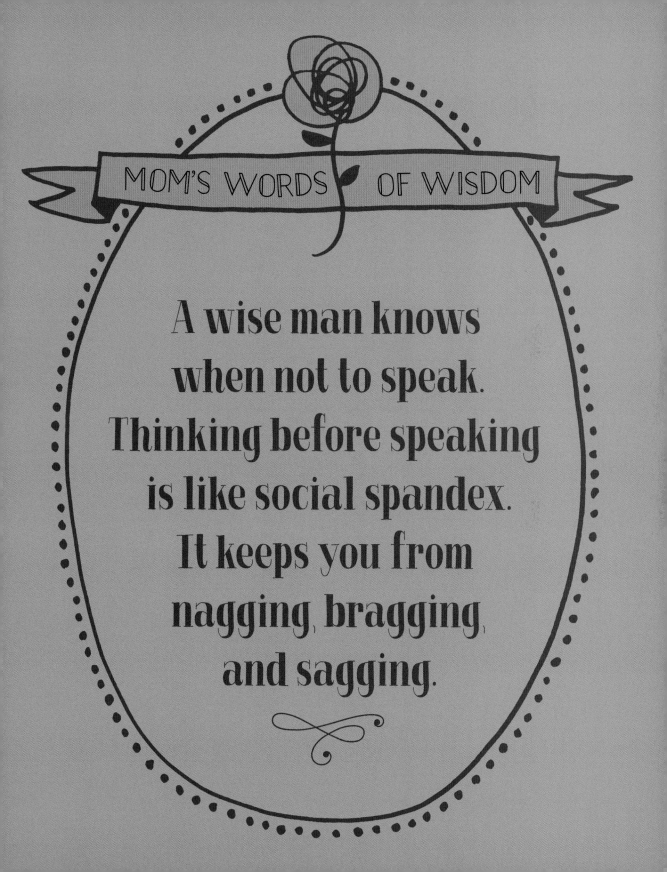

MOM'S WORDS OF WISDOM

A wise man knows
when not to speak.
Thinking before speaking
is like social spandex.
It keeps you from
nagging, bragging,
and sagging.

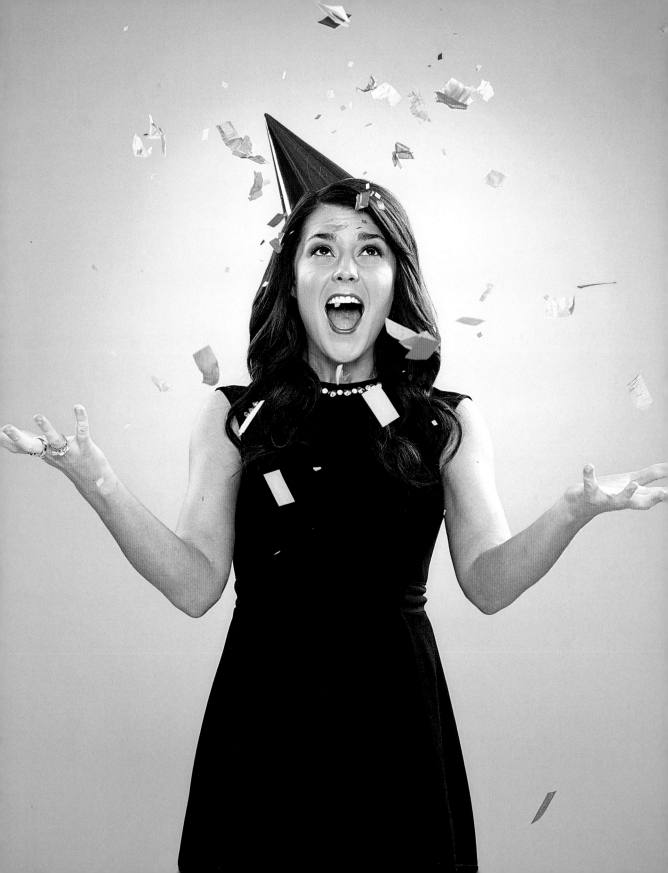

HOW TO THROW AN ADULT PARTY

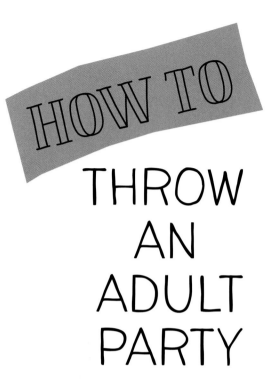

I'm still learning how to be a good hostess. When I was growing up, my parents hardly ever had friends over to our house and birthday parties were always sort of subdued, so I cultivated my party-hosting knowledge from TV, the Internet, and through the parties I've attended.

I lived in Brooklyn for almost five years, and in that time my roommates and I threw two *very* stupid parties. In NYC, it's more likely that you go out to a bar or restaurant with friends than hang out in someone's apartment. Space is limited and expensive and most of my friends were creative-types, so all of our apartments were kind of small and crappy and not conducive to parties.

But my two roommates and I still tried.

The apartment we were renting was abysmal, but it was in a cool neighborhood. We invited all of our comedy friends over and about twenty people dropped by. Our apartment had 1.5 bedrooms (one of my roommates slept in the living room) and it didn't have air-conditioning or a sink in the bathroom.

The three of us were completely used to this style of living and had forgotten that it wasn't normal or comfortable for others. We were quickly reminded when people had to wash their hands in our kitchen sink full of dirty dishes and Solo cups, and the living room instantly became hot and sweaty when occupied by more than three humans. Oops. We should have thought this through.

The night turned out okay, because everyone drank a lot more to mask their discomfort and we had roof access! HUZZAH! THERE IS A GOD! The party instantly transferred to the roof for the rest of the night and we were all finally able to air out our pits.

Here's a photo!

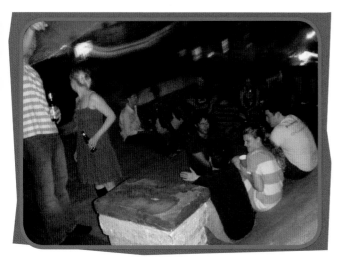

The next year, I moved into a separate place with one of my roommates, while the other roommate moved in with some Craigslist strangers (very nice strangers, though). The three of us decided we wanted to try to up our game and throw a *dinner* party in our slightly bigger, slightly nicer, OMG-there's-a-sink-in-the-bathroom apartment. *Dinner parties are what adults do*, we thought. *Let's get sophisticated.* But dinner requires food. Did any of us know how to cook? HUGE OVERSIGHT.

One of my roommates knew how to make really delicious scrambled eggs and the other knew how to make mashed potatoes and I knew how to buy hummus and pita chips. And that's what we did. We threw a very unsophisticated, confusing dinner party for about twenty to thirty people. But it was true to us. There was a tub of scrambled eggs and a tub of mashed potatoes and a tub of hummus and some other edible odds and ends and all the booze. It ended up

being a really fun time and I learned (the hard way) to never serve eggs at a party. Eesh.

Since then, I've been to a handful of really great house parties in New York and Los Angeles and I've slowly started to figure out what ingredients add up to prepping the primo partay. First step: don't call it a partay. And remember, at the end of the day it's about having a great time and making weird, egg-filled memories.

Food/Drink

Always have food and drinks.

A great party guest will bring some booze and/or food, but you should never assume people will do this. Also, I've found it's helpful to assume that all of your guests are depressed and miserable and then purchase party provisions with the mandate: *How can I make that chronically depressed person happy?* Think in a 360-degree way. Cups, vegan options, soda, Band-Aids, label what's in what cabinet and where the trash is, etc. What are all the possible things your guests could need or want to feel comfortable? I always try to put myself in the shoes of a visitor. When I go to someone else's house, what are my major stressors—other than the fact that I'm at a social event and that is very stressful to me? Oh, they have burgers *and* veggie burgers? This is a great party!

Invites

Send out invites.

Make sure people know. A party is a party when people are there. Who knew? Invite people directly—don't assume they'll see your Facebook event page or Instagram message or whatever method people use to pretend to communicate things in the future. I know you spent hours Photoshopping that hilarious-looking dog onto your kewl event poster, but also try texting and emailing to get the word out. That dog is pretty funny-looking, though.

pace

Make sure you have the space to accommodate human traffic.

This was the oversight with our first Brooklyn party. I'm naturally claustrophobic, so insert twenty friends into a tiny, air-conditioner-free apartment and you got yourself a panic-attack-themed party!

Try to invite the appropriate amount of people for the space you have. Not everyone you invite will come, but play it safe and assume all of your friends love you and have nothing better to do and will ALL come. Choose the space/number of guests to invite based on that.

Toilet Paper

ALWAYS HAVE MORE TOILET PAPER THAN NECESSARY.

And make it readily available for people to restock if necessary. One of the worst things in life, other than racism, is using the bathroom when the toilet paper has run out. It's a tragedy. Don't do that to your guests—stock up and store the TP in a place that's easy to access. Also, a match or a candle or some sort of spray is always handy if a guest has an "unexpected situation."

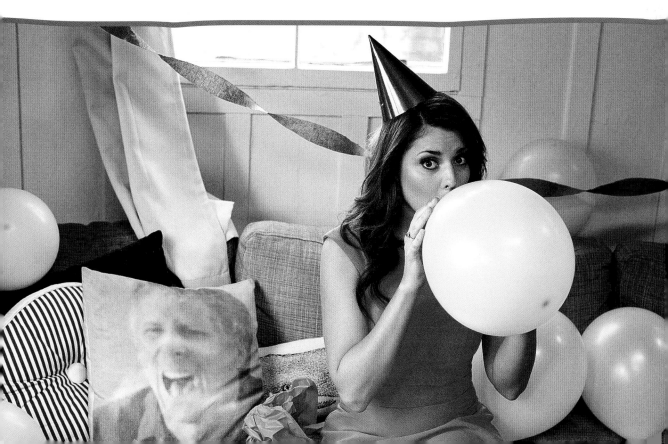

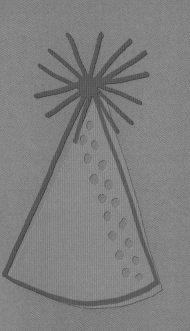

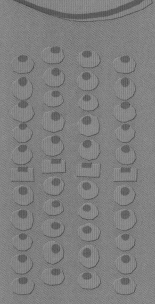

Background Music/ Entertainment

Create a nice ambience.

It's easier to talk when you subconsciously know that if there's a lull in the conversation there won't be complete silence. It feels like chatter. It can also serve as entertainment.

I went to a New Year's Eve party where a ten-second clip from the really dumb shower in *Starship Troopers* was played on a loop over the party music and it was hilarious. The more intoxicated everyone got, the more entrancing it was. Plus, it was a great conversation starter. Let's give 'em something to talk about.

Interesting Guests

Invite some wild cards.

It's always great to invite one or two people who either make great conversation or make for great conversation. They're the cream cheese that makes the human bagels more delicious. Yes, there's a chance they could go rogue and throw off the general vibe of the event, but they also might just make things more interesting. And parties are more fun when they're interesting.

Small Things

Love is in the details.

Pay attention to your guests during the party itself. Do they need a napkin? Who needs a chair? The little details make people think you're a thoughtful person. And that's cool because you are. Does Diane only drink red wine? Are there beer bottle openers? Is there a recycling can?

Do people know the trash is under the sink? Are there enough forks? And so on, and so fork.

Circulate

Make the rounds.

You invited all of these people, so give them the time of day and say something, anything, to as many as you can. Don't get stuck in one conversation all night. That's rude. Make everyone feel important and interesting. Give them the gift of conversation. Unless they're the type who don't want it. Then give them the gift of understanding their personal issues/space.

Unique Games/Themes

Games and theme parties bring everyone together.

A friend of mine used to throw a New Year's Eve party in Brooklyn every year that was FANTASTIC. He threw it six years in a row and every year it grew and people always looked forward to it. It was a pants-cutting party. Let me explain.

Each year he'd designate the "clothing theme" for everyone to wear. One year it was denim on denim, one year it was Barack Obama and Michael Jackson T-shirts and sweatpants, another year it was V-necks and pleated pants. Every half hour starting at nine p.m., everyone had to cut six inches off of his/her pants until midnight. But you weren't allowed to cut your own pants, someone else had to cut them for you. It made everyone interact with each other and it was so much fun *because* it was so off-the-wall stupid. Also, he had a giant pair of underwear that two people at a time could do shots in.

Potential **party games** (these are just some titles, you make of them what you will):

- Pants Cutting (Not my original game.)
- Throw This Thing into This Thing
- What's in This Dip?
- Will It Melt in the Microwave?
- Will This Shatter? (Only play this if the party is not in your abode.)
- Get Them Wet
- Make That Music Group Better (Name a popular band and see who you could sub into the band to make it better; for example, if you put Beyoncé in the Spice Girls they'd be better!)
- Scream Flip Cup (Play flip cup but scream while you try to flip your cup.)

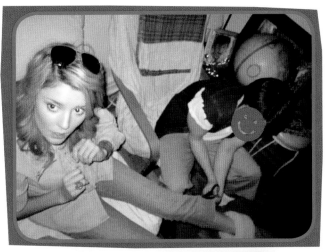

Ice

Always have ice.

It's a simple party luxury and a common after-thought, so take this tip as your reminder. Get ice. People like ice. Cold drinks are delicious.

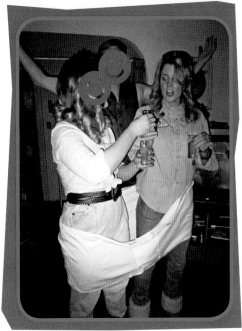

Transportation

TAKE ME HOME TONIGHT.

If it's possible to provide some sort of transportation for your guests, THAT WOULD BE EXCELLENT. You win.

This is less of a tip and more of a selfish dream I have to one day be driven to and from every party, so I never again have to wake up the next day and think, *Goddamn it, I have to go back to Mike's house to get my car. Please don't let his medium-hot roommate—who I spilled my rum and Coke all over—see me.*

GRACE'S GUIDE: CHANGING THE WORLD FOR THE BETTER. You're welcome.

Remember:

FIST BISCUIT

Food/Drink

Invites

Space

Toilet Paper

Background Music/
Entertainment

Interesting Guests

Small Things

Circulate

Unique Games/Themes

Ice

Transportation

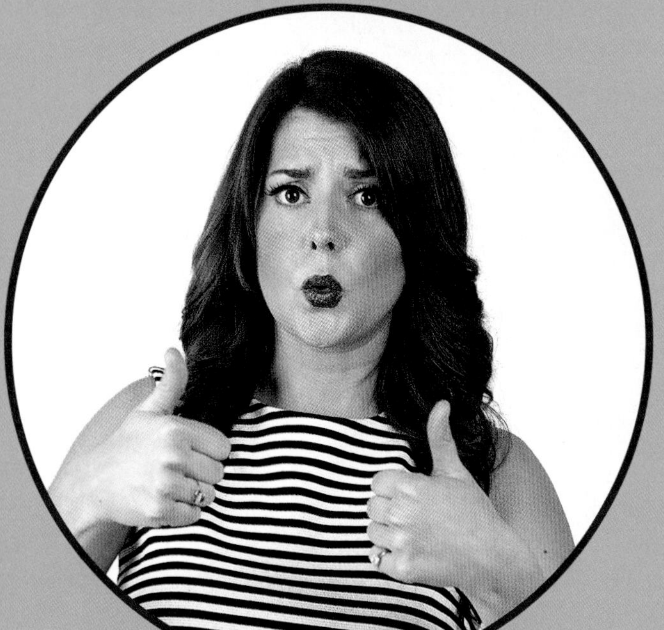

#FISTBISCUIT

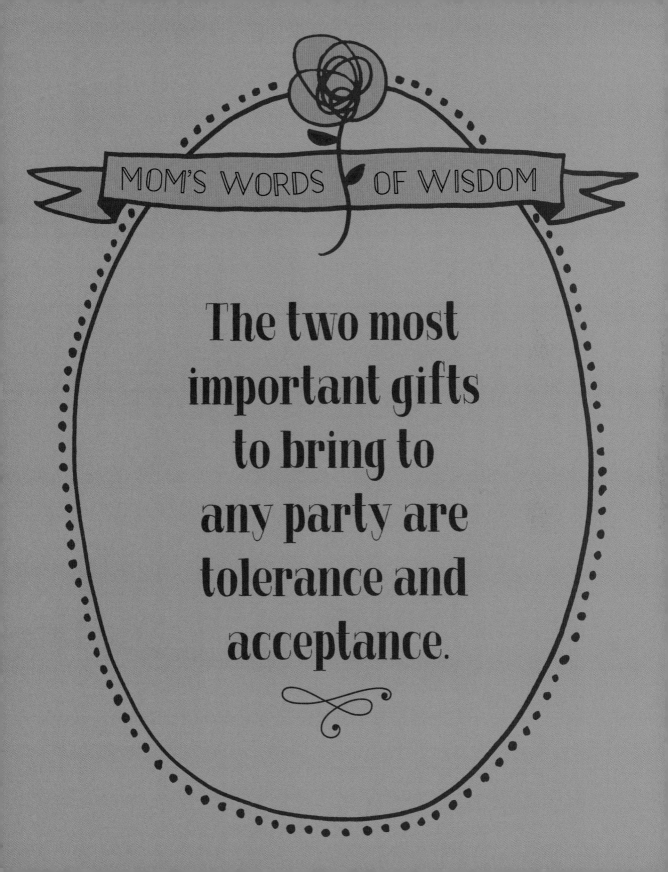

MOM'S WORDS OF WISDOM

The two most important gifts to bring to any party are tolerance and acceptance.

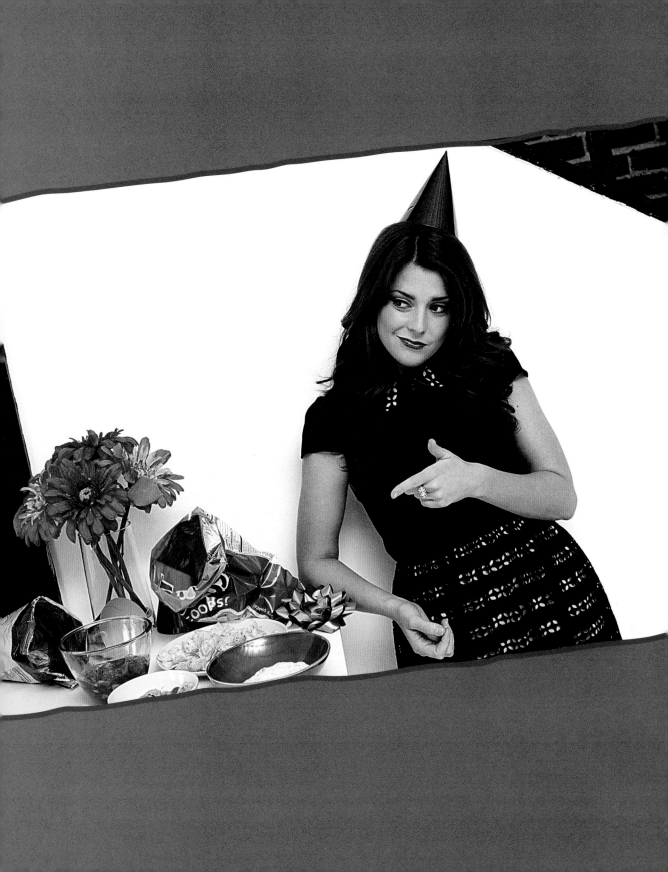

25

PARTY GUEST SURVIVAL TIPS

I hate parties. No, not true. I should say I hate the moments before I get to a party. Once I'm there and comfortable and a drink or three in, they're great. And afterward, I always feel good about myself that I went and interacted with other humans looking for fun. But for me, any planned social activity is preceded by hours and hours of internal debate about whether I should go or not. *What if I don't know more than one person there? What if I get stuck outside of conversation circles and have to look at my phone as if someone is desperately trying to get in touch with me, so I don't look socially stranded? WHAT IF MY PHONE DIES?*

I convince myself that it's fun to come up with excuses not to go to things. (Aaaaand, with that sentence, I will officially never be invited to any of my friends' or acquaintances' events ever again.) I get scared about being social. I've tried over the years to force myself into social situations so that

it becomes less of "a scary thing" and more of "a fun thing" to my brain.

For example, when I was supposed to meet my new boyfriend's friends for the first time, my flawed coping skills when it comes to social situations ruined everything. I had been dating this guy for a few months and thought he was the *coolest*, so clearly his friends had to be THE COOLEST, too. Oh god.

I had an improv show in Manhattan that night and I was going to meet up with them in Brooklyn as soon as it was done. I normally don't eat before shows due to my fear of losing control of my bowels onstage. When the show was over, I headed to the subway to get to Brooklyn. But before I got on I figured they'd all been drinking for hours ahead of me, so I should try to catch up. I bought three airplane-sized bottles of tequila before I got onto the subway and drank them in less than five minutes on an empty stomach.

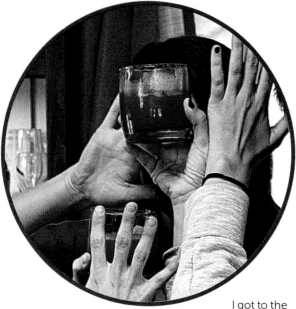

I got to the friend's apartment, and the night started out strong. I came in at the right time and we were all laughing and having fun. But two group beers and two group shots into the evening, everything faded to black for me. I was gone. The next thing I knew, it was the morning and I was puking into my boyfriend's toilet. I was twenty-four. I hadn't puked from drinking since I was seventeen. I found out later that a very sober friend (whom I had met for the first time that night) drove us home and for most of the ride I openly wept in the backseat while trying to open the car door to walk home. I'm very good at parties and social situations!

As years have gone by, I've learned more about myself and about the art of socializing. At the end of the day, if you do it right, it's great for you. Other humans are wonderful. It's one of the reasons we exist. I think. Or not. Maybe we exist as God's forever April Fool's joke. Either way, here are twenty-five tips that are helpful if you find yourself in the "party guest" scenario and aren't sure what to do.

1. **You're going.** This is happening. Don't let your brain consume itself with all of the excuses you could use to get out of it. Lord knows I do. Am I crazy? No, you are. You bought this book. Yes, it's fun to think of new ways to explain that your dog has diarrhea, but it's also fun once you get there to talk to other humans. Leave your dog's butthole alone.

2. **Don't dress to impress, dress to no-stress.** Find out as much information as you can about the "dress code" of this event/situation and dress to be in the solid fiftieth percentile. Don't go for the best- or worst-dressed list—go for the forgettable outfit. It won't stress you out as much.

3. **Assess what kind of drinking party this will be and formulate a game plan.** This applies to drinkers and nondrinkers alike. For drinkers: This is something that has ruined me in the past. Compare your personal tolerance against what you think will be the general consumption rate that evening and stay within your limits. For nondrinkers: Recognize when tolerance levels have been compromised and get out of there!

4. **Don't smell (at least try not to).** This is a general courtesy to other people. Get that deodorant ready.

5. **Don't get stuck in conversations near the bathroom.** One, you don't know what bodily functions/bodily FUN is happening in that room. Distance yourself. I find it's best to

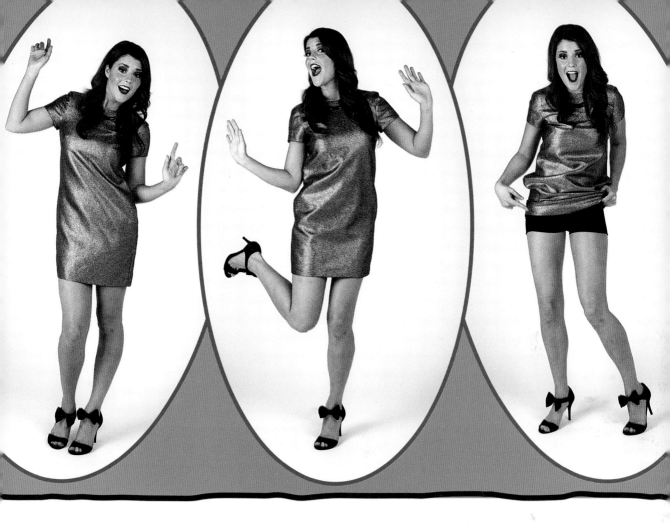

stay near an exit or window. It gives you something to look at if conversation lulls.

6. Let the conversations come to you.

In addition to #5, I find that sometimes it's best to plant yourself in a comfortable area of the room and let the conversations come to you. POWER MOVE. All of a sudden, you become an anchor and people want to know what's happening over there. Everyone seems to be coming and going from that corner. Hmm . . . social magnetism.

7. Don't be the #1 drunk or the date of the #1 drunk. I've gone to friends' weddings

before and been like, *No one knows me, I can drink and dance like no one is watching.* TURNS OUT EVERYONE IS WATCHING. If you're in a situation where you might run into/have to engage with more than 25 percent of the people there again *after* this event, I'd highly recommend keeping your cool and allowing someone else to win first place on this one.

8. Try to have conversations. Don't get

labeled as the person no one wants to talk to because you're impossible to engage. There always seems to be someone that everyone avoids talking to because it's more effort than it's

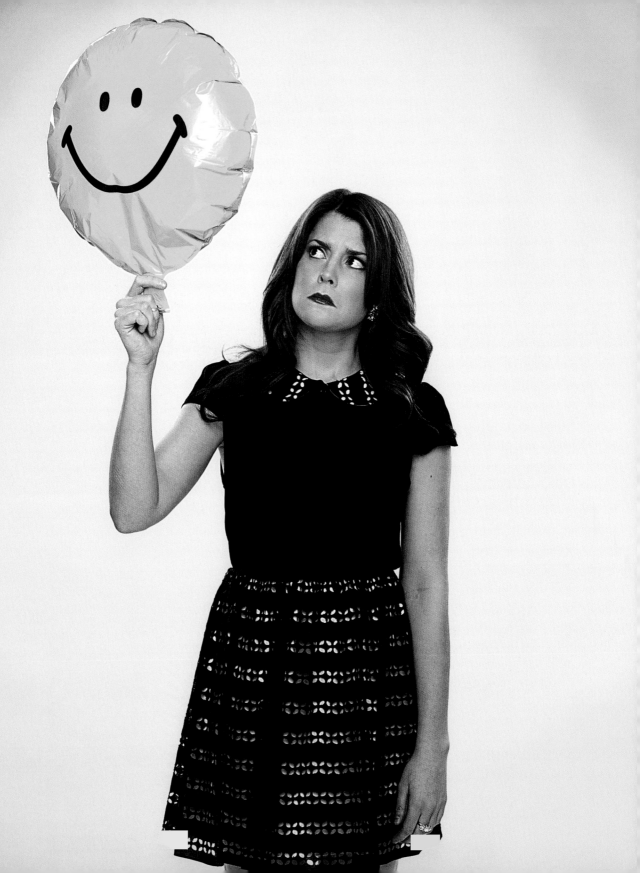

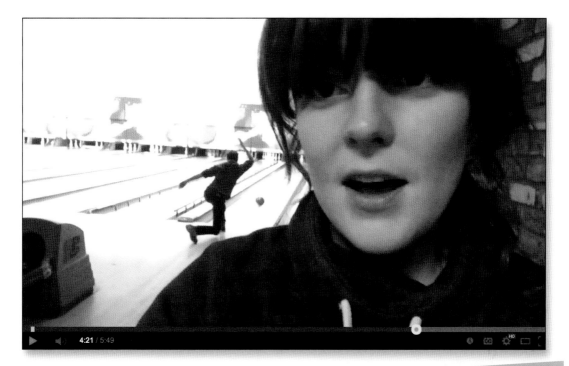

worth. If you find conversations hard, do what I do: ask questions! (See: sidebar on types of conversation starters.) Create conversation around the other person's answers! Yay! You're doing it!

9. **If there are less than a quarter of the attendees left at the party, it's probably time to leave.** Parties always reach a "max fun" point and then slowly dip into a "max weird" time. Leave when the meter is still in the fun zone.

10. **Get a party partner.** It's always best to experience parties with at least one other person who has your back. Try to go with someone whom you can rely on to get you out of there before either one of you swears you can do the "Oops . . . I Did it Again" dance for everyone and they're going to LOVE IT. And be a good partner back.

11. **I REPEAT: Make a pact with your party partner to get each other out of there before you make lasting mistakes.**

Potential conversation starters

1. I like your shoes; do you have any phobias?
2. What do you think you're allergic to that you don't already know about?
3. What do you do for a living? LOL, sike, I don't care. Farting on a plane is the best, right?
4. What was the last thing you ate?
5. What type of piñata do you most prefer hitting?
6. Have you ever spent time in a bowling alley in the afternoon on a weekday? It's weird.
7. Do you have more pairs of underwear than you have cousins?
8. What animal would you most like to push into a giant cake?
9. If you could rename "toes," what would you call them?
10. What do you think is the worst tattoo imaginable?

We live in a plugged-in world. Unfortunately, you can't get away with puking in a skillet anymore without it becoming a viral video. So get ready for your new career, unless you find a savvy party partner.

12. Go for the hug. When saying good-bye, it's best to keep your hands out and assume it's a hug. If they're for sure going for the handshake, then re-adjust. You don't want to be the guest who's inebriated or saying good-bye to an inebriated person and you half commit to a handshake and then realize they're going in for the hug and before you know it your hand is accidentally stroking a crotch.

13. Beware of group punches/jungle juices. They can sneak up on you. Drinking out of troughs in general—unless you're at a frat/sorority party or you're actually a farm pig who can handle liquor (PIGS, DON'T DO IT!)—should be approached with caution. Especially when you're a party guest. My general rule of thumb for party liquids is: bring the beverage you want to drink to the party.

14. Bring something! Food, booze, and/or a gift. Even if it's for you (see #13 about bringing your own beverage). This is a sign of goodwill and makes you look like you care about other people. You're one of the three wise men. And they never even RSVP'd.

15. You don't HAVE to eat the food. Especially if you know your body probably won't handle it properly. If you're on the fence about it, bunt and play it safe. Don't bet on your bowels. It's ALWAYS better to politely pass on the food than to politely pass gas in the corner.

16. Don't take a dump in the guest bathroom (see #15).

17. Help the host. (I AM THE ABSOLUTE WORST AT THIS.)

18. Don't hover near the dips. Get away from the food table after snacking. When conversations get stuck there, it can be less than fun. You open yourself up to not only a new world of awkward conversations, but also new, awkward conversations with spinach dip in between everyone's teeth.

19. **Don't get stuck with the pet.** The party pet is a lot like your phone. When no one is talking to you, you can rely on the pet, because it doesn't have any sexts to respond to. But as a pseudo-adult, you shouldn't spend more than one-quarter of the party with the pet. That seems normal and fun and less weird.

20. **Be gracious and say good-bye.** Unless you're not capable of saying good-bye without embarrassing yourself. Then you should IRISH GOOD-BYE. See the "How to Do the Walk of Shame" chapter for more information on Irish Good-byes.

21. **Don't get caught up in gossip.** You can listen, but don't overindulge.

22. **Participate in games.** Why not?

23. **Don't be racist/homophobic (overall life tip).**

24. **Know how you're getting home.** Is your friend taking you? Are you cabbing it? Are you leaving your car? If so, where? Make a plan in advance—it will alleviate A TON of stress before, during, and (the morning) after the party.

25. **YOU DID IT—CONGRATULATE YOURSELF!**

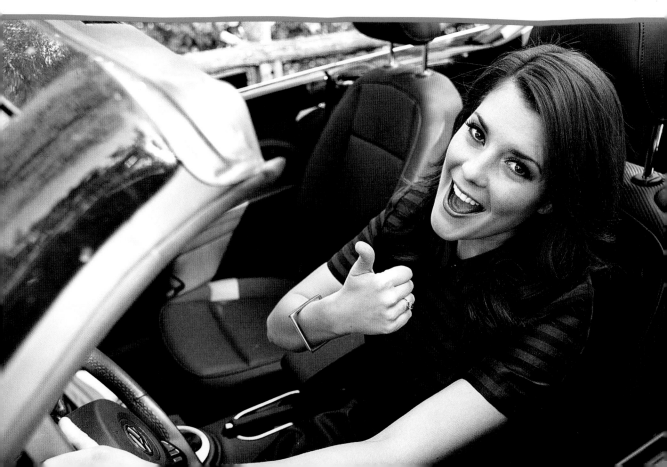

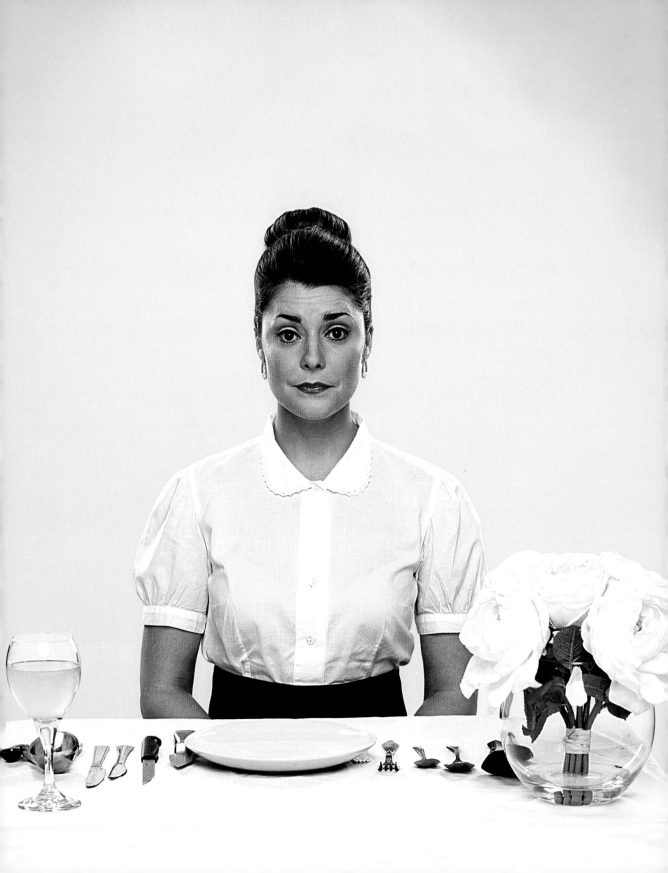

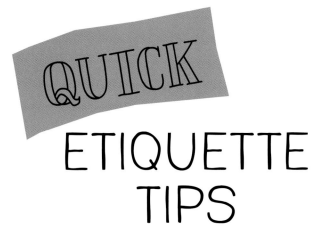

QUICK ETIQUETTE TIPS

Saying the right thing at the right time is difficult. It's like playing Jenga blindfolded. You make a choice and hope you build the tower up instead of knocking it down. Eep.

Having something helpful to say when some major unexpected life event strikes is a really great thing to have in your back pocket.

PAUSE. ANECDOTE TIME.

I was recommended a dog-walker through a friend, and when I met him for the first time I realized he was truly a dog person. He came to my place on a Saturday soaking wet because he spent that morning teaching a couple dachshunds how to swim in a nearby lake. I instantly hired him to walk my dog a few days a week.

My dog is extremely aggressive and trusts no one, and he walked her for weeks. She loved him and ended up getting along really well with all of the other dogs he brought on walks, which

was *so rare*. LIFE IS GREAT! GETTING THIS DOG WASN'T A MISTAKE.

And then things took a turn. The dog-walker called me and said he needed to talk. I found out from a friend who also hired him to walk her dog that he had suddenly decided to quit the dog-walking business. WHAT? The guy who spent every waking hour of his day loving dogs was quitting the dog business? How and why and WHAT?

It took me two days to build up the courage to call him back. He told me he was quitting the dog-walking business because the week prior his own dog was attacked on a walk by a client's dog, which he'd been walking peacefully together with his dog for years. He had to rush his dog to the vet and four days later the dog died. He said it changed his entire view of dogs and it was too hard for him to be around them.

WHOA.

I tried to console him to the best of my abilities. Which included me saying the phrase "Oh, man" on repeat. He clearly wanted someone to talk to, because he stayed on the phone with me for almost an hour explaining his pain as I replied, "Oh, man," "I'm so sorry," and "Wow." The conversation was weirdly personal but ended on a hopeful note when he asked me how I made money on YouTube, because he was interested in pursuing it as a new career option. If you happen to see a dog whisperer from the Valley on YouTube, send him my regards.

But that conversation is a great example of the types of interpersonal conversations that could present themselves at any point. Here are some examples of good versus bad things to say when a human you do or don't know approaches you with struggles.

THE STRUGGLE:
My Family Member Died

Things Not to Say:
- I can relate, I killed my toilet earlier.
- Same! My family member dyed . . . their hair yesterday.
- I finally watched *Breaking Bad*, so good.

Things to Say:
- I know everyone is telling you they're sorry, I honestly don't know what to say exactly, but I want you to know I'm here for you.
- This sucks a dick.
- I'm going to leave you alone, unless you want me near, I love you.

THE STRUGGLE:
I Just Got Dumped

Things Not to Say:
- I just took a dump! Oh wait, you said something different.
- Dumps like a truck, what what. I love "The Thong Song"!
- I also hate Donald Trump.

Things to Say:
- This moment feels like the worst, which means things are about to get better.
- Feel sad and bummed and wild for however long it takes.
- I bought you a gift.

THE STRUGGLE:
I Got Fired

Things Not to Say:
- I can relate . . . *lights a candle*
- I adopted three redheaded orphans. I just wanted you to feel better.
- I puked inside a duck's mouth. By accident.

Things to Say:
- Yes! Congratulations, this job was awful!!
- Shhh-shhh-shhhh, here's another margarita.
- I puked inside a duck's mouth. By accident.

THE STRUGGLE:
I'm Pregnant

Things Not to Say:
- I know a place . . .
- I'm so sorry.
- YOU GON GET FAAAAAT.

Things to Say:
- Congratulations, you're going to be a wonderful parent.
- Can I babysit?
- What type of pickles do you like best?

THE STRUGGLE:
We're Getting Married

Things Not to Say:
- Well then, I guess I won't be needing this engagement ring anymore. So much for my dreams of a viral wedding proposal video . . . *turns off hidden camera* Tell the marching band they can go home.
- Why?
- Eesh. Good luck. Yowch. Woof. Tough one. Oof. You had such potential. Well, one of you did.

Things to Say:
- YAY! Where's the champagne?
- This is great news! How can I help?
- You can use my dog/adorable child as a ring bearer if you want.

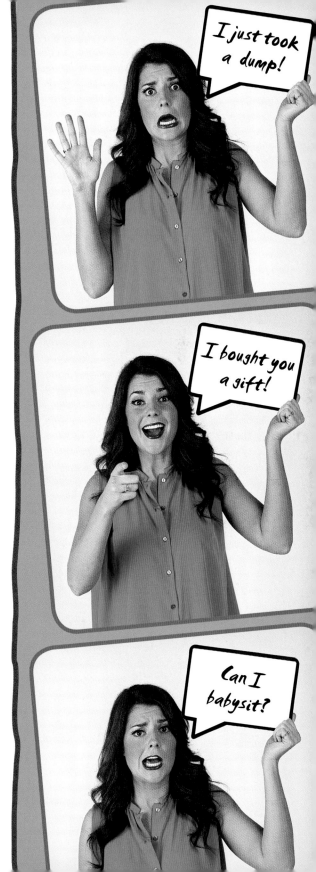

THE ART OF NOT DYING ALONE

THE ART OF TRUSTING
SOMEONE TO TOUCH
MOUTHS WITH YOU

THE ART OF BEING A WHIRLING DERVISH
OF VULNERABILITY

THE ART OF BEING BOTH
THE HAPPIEST AND SADDEST
YOU'VE EVER BEEN

THE ART OF GETTING A DECENT FREE MEAL

THE ART OF ATTRACTION,
COMMITMENT, AND WAKING UP WITH
THE LEAST AMOUNT OF REGRET

The Art of PUTTING Yourself OUT There

~~THE ART OF FINDING THE RIGHT PERSON TO KISS YOU INSIDE THE MOUTH~~

~~THE ART OF LETTING SOMEONE INTO YOUR PRIVATE(S) LIFE~~

~~THE ART OF ATTRACTION, REJECTION, RINSING AND REPEATING~~

Your Love Life

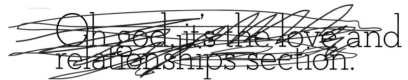
Oh god, it's the love and relationships section.

Oh god, it's the love and relationships section. I can hear your private parts sighing. What do I have to say about relationships, and what possible advice could I give you? This is the one part of my life that I try to keep offline. I trick myself into thinking it gives me balance to have one thing that's just for me.

BUT NOT TODAY! Today, I'll let you in on some private stuff. Ah, geez. I can already taste the regret. It tastes like coffee. Oh wait, that's my coffee. It tastes like bacon. No, wait, sorry, that's my plate of bacon. Yes, I'm eating a plate of just bacon. Stalling . . . now let's talk about relationships!

I met my first high school boyfriend at a Latin convention in Kentucky the summer before my junior year.

PAUSE. Did I just say Latin convention?

Here's the thing: In high school I was a pseudo-nerd. I wasn't smart enough about physics or anime to be a full-fledged nerd, but I also wasn't cool enough to be one of the popular kids who were into drugs and music. I was in what I like to call nerd purgatory. So I attended things like Latin conventions, which were weeklong conventions for horny, socially awkward, slightly to grossly above-average high school students who wanted an excuse to hang out with other horny, kind-of-smart kids from around the country, under the guise that it was for academic purposes.

The conventions were held at college campuses, so we got to sleep in co-ed dorms and it felt SO SCANDALOUS. There were a lot of activities throughout the week—both athletic and academic. And every night there was a dance, where we got to release some of our horny energy via casual, awkward grinding.

I initially decided to go to this convention because a couple of my Latin Club girlfriends (I'M STILL SUCH A PSUEDO-NERD) had attended the year before and had so much fun making out with "hot dudes." We were representing Jersey, after all, so as nerdy as we were, there was still some trashy sex appeal to us.

When we got to the convention, we set our sights on the guys hailing from the all-boys school in Wisconsin. They were upper middle class, handsome, well read, and had nothing to lose (their high school was like a pre-Harvard—they were all going to be fine).

One of my friends went after the boy that I wanted—the cute, not gay, fun-loving, smart one. So instead I fixed my sights on the tall, blond, older, handsome one. We flirted and grinded (I'm so bad at grinding—the main thing that I learned at the convention) all week, and near the end I found out he had a girlfriend. WHAT A WONDERFUL DISCOVERY. My horniness deflated like a sad week-old birthday balloon.

I rebooted my system and was set to find another Wisconsin boy (after all, they were the Nordstrom's to our Hot Topic) but at the last dance (the one that counts because everyone is SUPER desperate) none of them were there. We later learned that they had all gotten kicked out of the convention because they were caught drinking. That's why they were so full of life! They were bad boys! Uh-oh, I liked that.

After the convention my "Latin girlfriend" had gone back to the Jersey dude she was already talking to and stopped talking to the Wisconsin boy that I wanted. One night, I grew some digital testicles and IM'd him. It worked. We had an effortlessly fun conversation and started chatting regularly on IM (instant messenger—even back then

I was ahead of the curve with Internet dating). Turns out we had a lot in common and made each other "LOL" (when LOL wasn't cliché).

Before we knew it, my Midwest Mister and I were talking to each other every day after school for hours. We compared our days, and did some heavy Internet flirting (not cybering, you pervs). Eventually we considered ourselves to be "dating," whatever that meant. All I knew was that the guys in my Jersey high school couldn't compare to my wonderful Wisconsin sort-of-boyfriend.

I didn't really talk to my parents about my love life back then. That all changed the day my dad took me to Best Buy so I could buy a Ben Folds CD, because my secret Badger State BF had recommended it. God, we were so white.

When my dad asked me how I had heard of Ben Folds, I ended up telling him about my cheesehead Romeo. It was the first time I had ever mentioned a crush to my dad (I'm pretty sure he was starting to believe I was into the V). There was a pause in conversation and my dad finally said, "Why don't you go out there and see him?"

WHAT? TURNS OUT DAD IS HAPPY I'M INTO THE D.

Next thing I knew, my stepmom and I were on a plane out to Wisconsin so I could go to prom with Mr. Milwaukee. I don't know if the trip was better for me or for my stepmom. It was definitely her Cinderella moment—except in this version the stepmom is SUPER COOL. But overall, it was a great weekend. His family was the picture of Midwest charm and hospitality. His parents were still married (da fuq?).

The prom was in a beautiful museum and I got to be the Mysterious Girlfriend from Out of Town That No One Knows and Can Have Any Crazy Adventurous Super Cool Backstory. And then we made out in a car for a couple of hours. Neat.

Over the next year, my all-boys-school sweetheart and I visited each other a few more times and exchanged thousands of instant messages. Eventually it fizzled out as I got ready for college and started to look for boys IRL. However, we still check in with each other from time to time over Facebook (aka I have some drinks and look through his photos—good times).

Why did I tell you this story? Hmm, excellent question. To prove I made out with someone once . . . ?

S l o w l y sashays away to the bathroom

AND I'M BACK.

Young love is so ridiculous, as is middle-aged and old love. And it's also

hilarious. When have you ever felt so vulnerable and wonderful and terrible at the same time? Maybe in a pole-dancing class?

Trying to find true love is a daunting, annoying, and seemingly impossible task, especially now that everyone is so plugged in. Thanks to social media and search engines, you can find out a lot of random information—too much—about a person before ever meeting them. I'm learning new stuff about myself via the Internet every day. For instance, I played a process server on a "reality show" for truTV in 2010. I had conveniently forgotten about this until the Internet reminded me the other day. Fun!

But finding someone special in this .gif-able world is possible. Love is a battlefield, as Pat Benatar once said. And we should all be prepared.

Allow me to try to suit you up for battle (emphasis on "try").

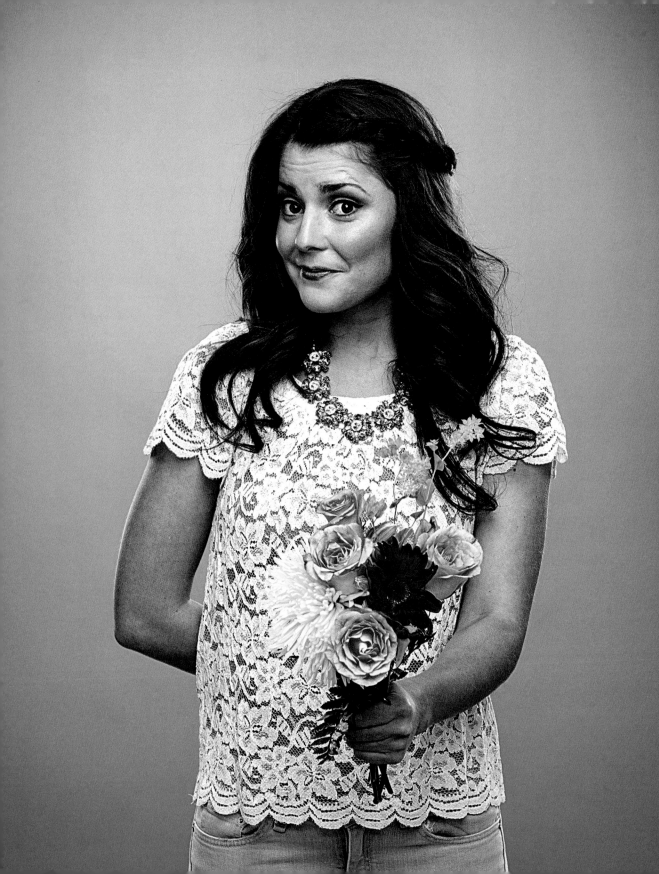

HOW TO ASK SOMEONE OUT

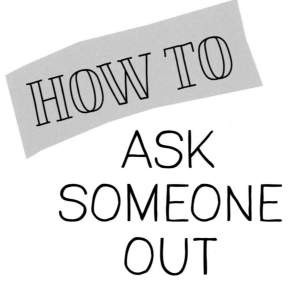

Asking someone out is one of the most vulnerable experiences in life. You might as well walk up to the person in question completely nude and say, "Does this appeal to you?" Don't do that. You could get arrested.

I don't have a lot of experience asking people out. I'm a serial-monogamous-relationship type and when I do "flirt" with someone or organize some sort of date/meeting, I usually rely on technology to help. I'M WEAK AND SCARED OF REJECTION, OKAY? So I'm the perfect human to give you advice on putting yourself out there. Smiley face emoticon.

But I have been asked out (believe it or not) and I've helped friends and Internet strangers alike ask other people out. I've made Web videos to help unknown Internet users ask girls and guys to proms and I've even helped with marriage proposals.

Here's an example of what NOT to do. One time I was wearing a horizontal-striped shirt in a bar and a guy said to me, "You must have a lot of confidence." I said, "Why do you say that?" And he said, "Because horizontal stripes make a girl look fat." And I thought to myself, not only do I need this man's number so I can hire him to be my future stylist, but I need his number so I can call him every morning and remind him not to say sh*t like that to girls ever.

He was negging, and negging is stupid (and trust me, I'm not negging you by saying that). "Negging" is a term invented by *The Pickup Artist* and according to Urban Dictionary it means: "Low-grade insults meant to undermine the self-confidence of a woman so she might be more vulnerable to your advances."

It's as dumb as having a wiener on your forehead.

I've devised what I think is a solid method for asking someone on a date. But before we get into this, remember that what you're doing is cool. You're putting yourself out there, because you want love and companionship. You're not a serial killer! And that's a neat thing to discover about yourself.

Decide

Make the choice.

And be steadfast. (Not to be confused with Stedman—though he also made a choice. But did he? I feel like a choice was made for him. Stop it, Grace. You already spend too much time thinking about Stedman.) You're going to ask [insert name of the person who makes your privates feel weird] on a date. It's happening. Yes. Don't have second thoughts about it. You might not be the most confident person, but at least you'll have confidence in this decision. And that's exciting. You're about to do something terrifying.

YES. I truly believe that when we do things that scare us, even if they turn out poorly, they help us grow. Except for swimming with sharks or holding snakes. Nothing about that will help me grow. People who swim with sharks are dumb. Unless they're scientists and they're studying them to help the world on some level. Then that's cool, I guess. But to swim with them for fun? Get real.

Imagine

Imagine the worst-case scenario.

I used to do competitive gymnastics for a brief moment in time from fifth through eighth grade. I was stunted in my growth back then. Ah, those were the days. My coaches used to tell us to visualize our routines. Picture yourself doing the flip,

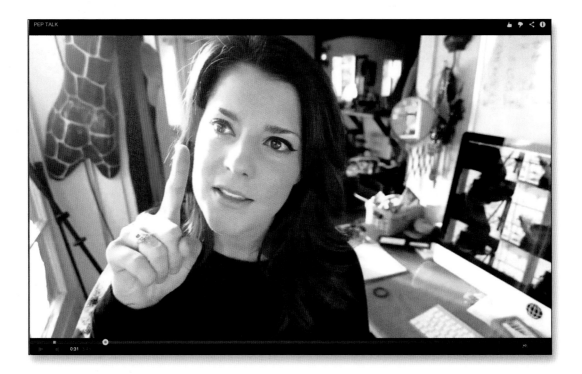

PEP TALK

0:31

release, twist, etc., in your mind. Imagine it happening perfectly and your body will follow.

That never happened for me. My brain would imagine it and my body wouldn't always do it. As I got older, auditioning for TV, film, commercials, and performing live improv and sketch comedy, I would try to imagine myself nailing the audition or show and most of the time it didn't go that way.

Instead, I started imagining the worst-case scenarios. I imagined myself throwing up on casting directors at the very end of my laxative commercial audition, sh*tting my pants in the middle of an improv scene about my laxative not working, and falling out of my chair and splitting my head open on the set of *Chelsea Lately* before they cut to the laxative commercial I never booked.

Once I started imagining terrible scenarios, things started to improve. For some complex psychological reason, letting the worst possible scenario play out in my head took the gravity out of the situation.

My friend Mamrie, who is an amazing sketch comedy performer, always says to herself before she goes onstage, *If you sh*t your pants onstage, you can always move back to North Carolina and start a new life.*

I really believe that acknowledging the worst possible thing that can happen frees you from the fear of it. So before you ask your dreamboat on a date, imagine it going terribly wrong. And then imagine it going terribly in another way. If you can do a better job in real life than your two nightmare scenarios, then you've succeeded—even if they say no.

Make Peace
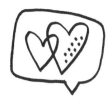

Make peace with failure.

It's possible that the person you ask won't give you the answer that you're hoping for. That's okay. Allow yourself to recognize "no" as a possible outcome. Try searching "wedding proposals gone awry" on YouTube. I don't say this to deter you, but to allow you to see the flip side.

I've always had the mind-set of going into a situation with slightly lower expectations/standards and then letting myself be pleasantly surprised. Don't set yourself up for failure—just make peace with it as a possible outcome. It might give you more confidence to acknowledge that this could end with rejection. I HATE to reference "YOLO" . . . so I won't. Just know we're all going to die someday and it's better to have tried and failed than never to have tried at all.

Plan

Make a plan. Get prepared.

Approach the situation like you would an earthquake or a zombie apocalypse. If you don't have plans for earthquakes or zombie apocalypses, that's cool. Just watch any show on TLC and you'll get some inspiration. However, don't watch TLC to get dating inspiration. They literally have a show about women going to each other's weddings just to talk smack about every element of it. Then they vote on who threw the best wedding (aside from their own, of course). Oh, The Learning Channel.

Anyway, you should have a solid(ish) plan of attack for how you'll be making the approach.

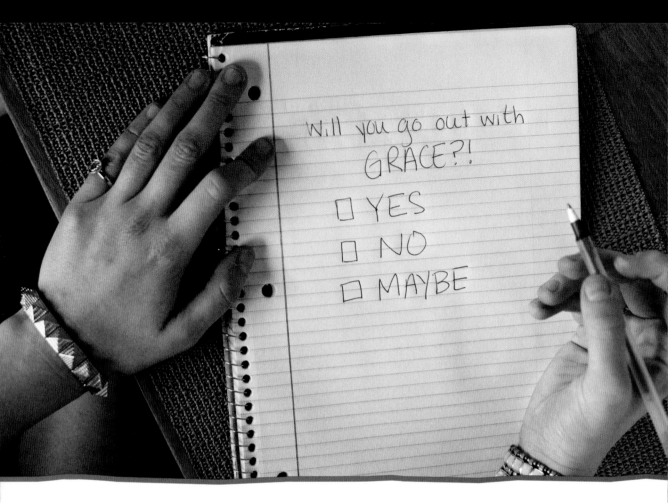

Will it be by phone? In person? Over email? Will it happen between classes? Through mutual friends? After a party? Try to be as clear as you can, so things can happen as smoothly as possible. But remember, it's also nice for spontaneity to play a part, so don't be discouraged if things don't go exactly as planned. Be ready, willing, and open. Like a prostitute.

ie

Lie to your confidence.

Not to the person you're about to ask out. Don't do that. Instead, lie to your confidence and pretend that you're not afraid of what you're about to do. You got this. You're a champion, a hero,

an organ donor, etc. Pump yourself up and get excited. You're about to play some emotional sport and you've been (kind of) training for this moment. Your heart is Rocky and the other person is the stairs. Google it. CLEAR EYES, FULL HEART, CAN'T LOSE. Except when you lose. True story, that's the chant my improv team would scream before we went onstage.

Before I do anything I'm afraid of, I listen to some sweet, sweet *Jock Jams*. Unfortunately for me, listening to *Jock Jams* has never been ironic. Everyone has their own method of getting themselves amped up (god, I feel like I'm selling you an energy drink), so find yours. Tell yourself you can do this. Remember, if you fail you can start a new life for yourself in North Carolina.

Enjoy

Enjoy yourself!

Or at least try to. If you're having fun, you'll probably get a better reaction from your prey/future-potential date. They say laughter is infectious; I like to think positive energy is, too. And it's great for your potential dates to know that the only thing they'll contract from you is a great attitude (I'll take my chlamydia on the side, please).

Have you ever watched a standup comedian or a musician who's really, really enjoying herself onstage? It's great! I remember seeing the band Matt and Kim for the first time at a festival in upstate New York four years ago. Kim played the drums with a huge smile on her face during THE WHOLE SHOW. And I loved it! I was so mesmerized by their charisma. Also, I had a huge crush on Matt and then interviewed them afterward, only to find out that they were a couple. But they were such a happy couple that I couldn't help but admire their relationship.

The same goes for that viral video of the guy dancing by himself at the Sasquatch! Music Festival. He's having a hilariously great time all alone and eventually hundreds of people swarm his area and it becomes a massive dance party. His energy is infectious.

Positive energy persuades people. Don't let potential dates turn you down because you weren't enthusiastic. Let them turn you down because of the chlamydia.

Funny

A sense of humor can be a lethal weapon.

I'm not saying go up to your date with the opening line, "Knock, knock. Who's there? Me. I'll always be here for you. Will you go out with me?" Sweet Jesus, no. But humor can take a lot of the pressure off the askee. And, personally, I think having a sense of humor is one of the most attractive qualities in a person. And I think everyone else in the world shares my specific beliefs, so you should take this very, very seriously.

Here are a couple pick-up lines for you that are so over-the-top stupid that your future partner won't be able to help but laugh at them (hopefully, unless they're terrible humans).

- You're like a fine wine. I don't know where you came from, you're hard to open, and you leave a metallic taste in my mouth.
- Look, I'm not a cashier but I've been CHECKing you out.

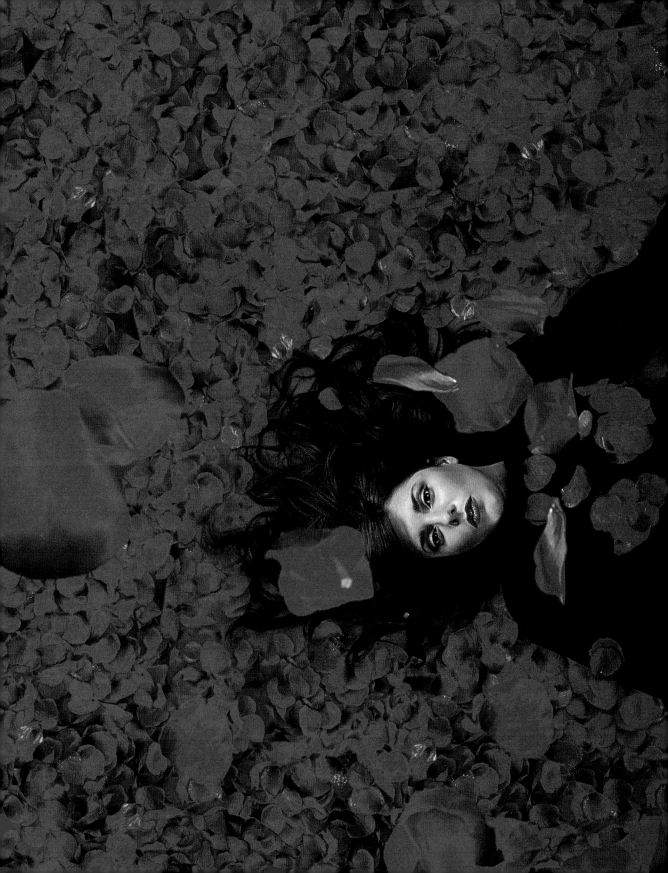

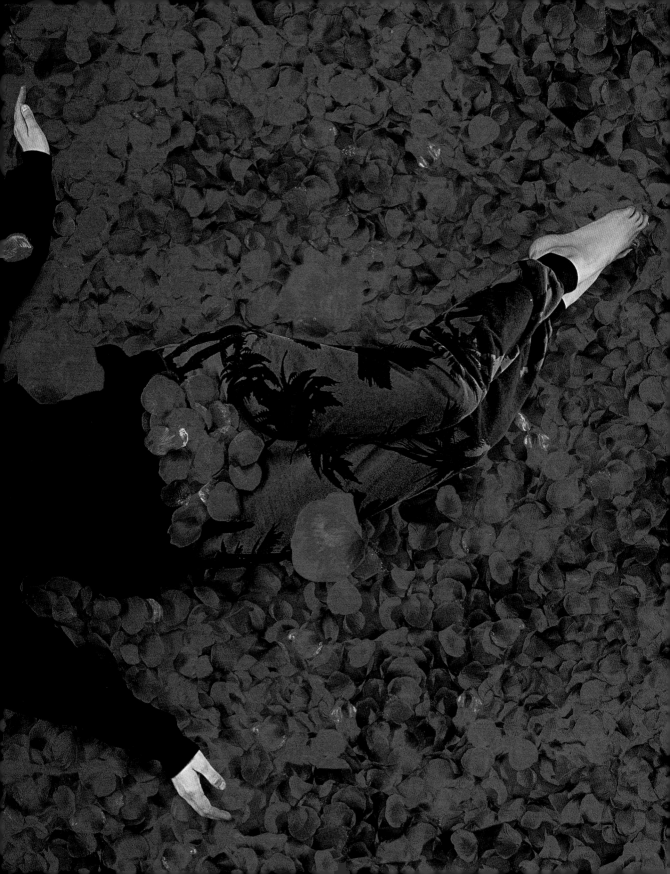

- (for Internet daters) Do you believe in love at first site?
- Is your name Instagram? Because I'd double-tap that.
- Just call me the garbage man because I always bag it up. #recycle
- Are you tired? Because you've been doing a sensible mix of yoga and weight-training in my head all day.
- Roses are red. Violets are blue. I have a high-functioning brain. Will you go out with me?

Attempt

Now is the time to go for it.

Whether it's over email, in person, or on some other social media platform, it's do or die. You won't die. So just do it. Go for it and don't look back. Unless there's someone stalking you. Then look back and call the cops. Otherwise do it!

Ask! Go! Go! Go! You can do this! I BELIEVE IN YOU. This section isn't so much informative as it is me yelling at you to do it. DO IT.

Look in the mirror and say to yourself, "Why don't we call gloves hand-shoes?" and then say to yourself, "You can do this." Be positive, be light, be yourself. Don't overanalyze, just get it over with. By this point you should probably stop reading this section and JUST DO IT.

-it

Aka exit!

Don't linger too long after you get your answer. Whether it's in real life, text life, email life, etc., let the conversation come to an end, so it can pick back up again on the actual date. Or if they say no, let it go and save face.

This part is kind of hard, because if they say yes, it's natural to want to keep the positive energy flowing, but save something for the date. Usain Bolt doesn't blow his load on preliminaries. Go for the gold.

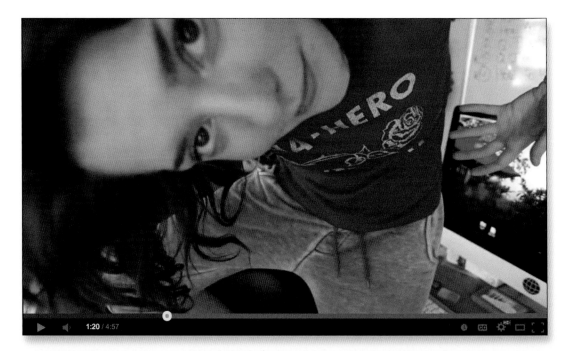

Remember: **DIMPLE FAX**

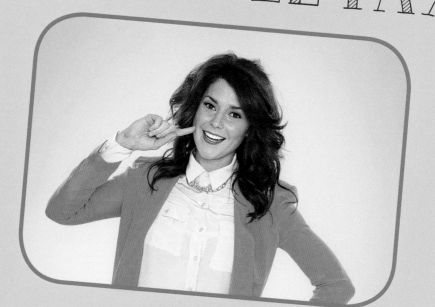

Decide
Imagine
Make peace
Plan
Lie
Enjoy

Funny
Attempt
X-it

#DIMPLEFAX

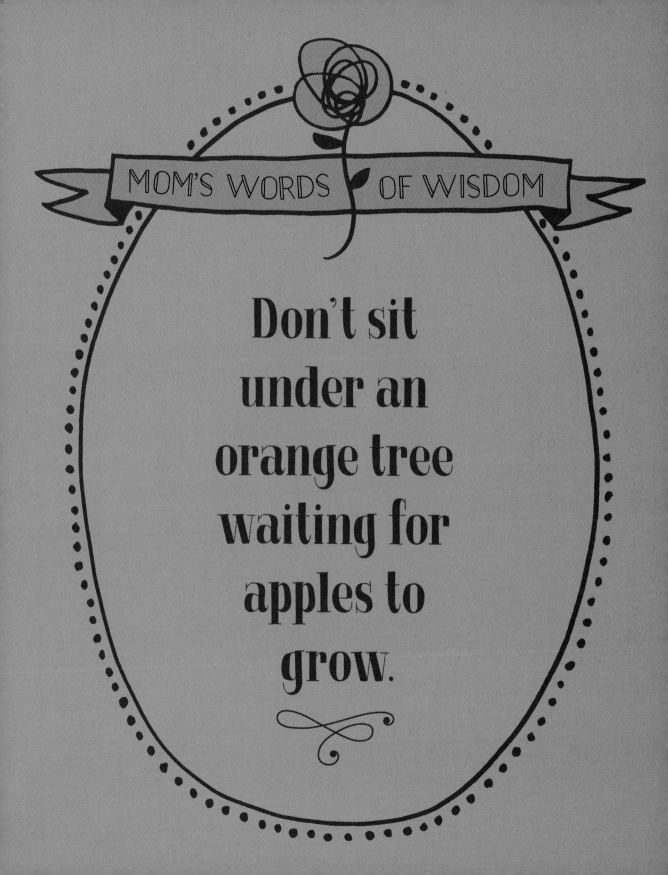

MOM'S WORDS OF WISDOM

Don't sit under an orange tree waiting for apples to grow.

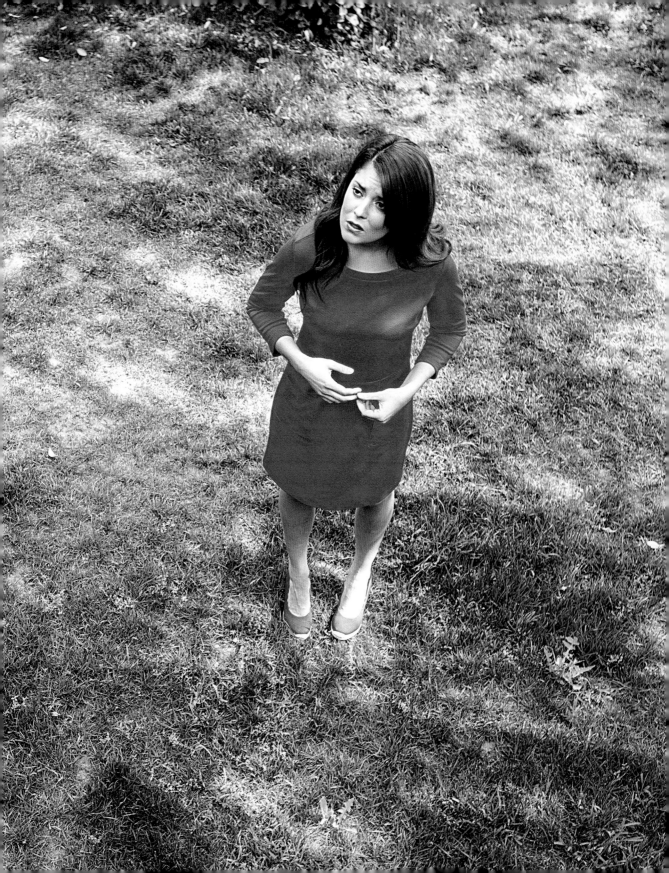

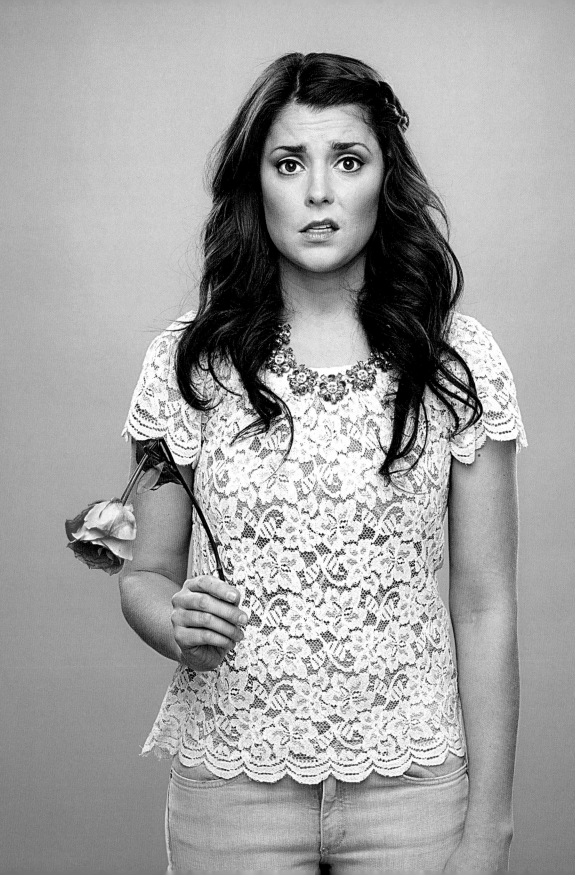

HOW TO ASK SOMEONE OUT

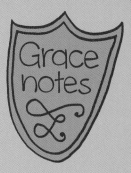

List three of the **WORST** possible outcomes for the situation (for example, you're bold and decide to wear white pants and your bowels are also bold and decide to make an unanticipated appearance outside your body):

1. _____
2. _____
3. _____

List three of the **WORST** things that have ever happened to you in your whole life:

1. _____
2. _____
3. _____

Whoa, that's some terrible stuff. Sorry, dude.

List three of the **WORST** things that have happened in the history of the world (feel free to Google search):

1. _____
2. _____
3. _____

YIKES! OUR WORLD IS MESSED UP. Now asking someone out doesn't seem so bad, right? If it still sounds terrifying, I drew this picture for you:

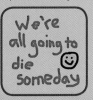

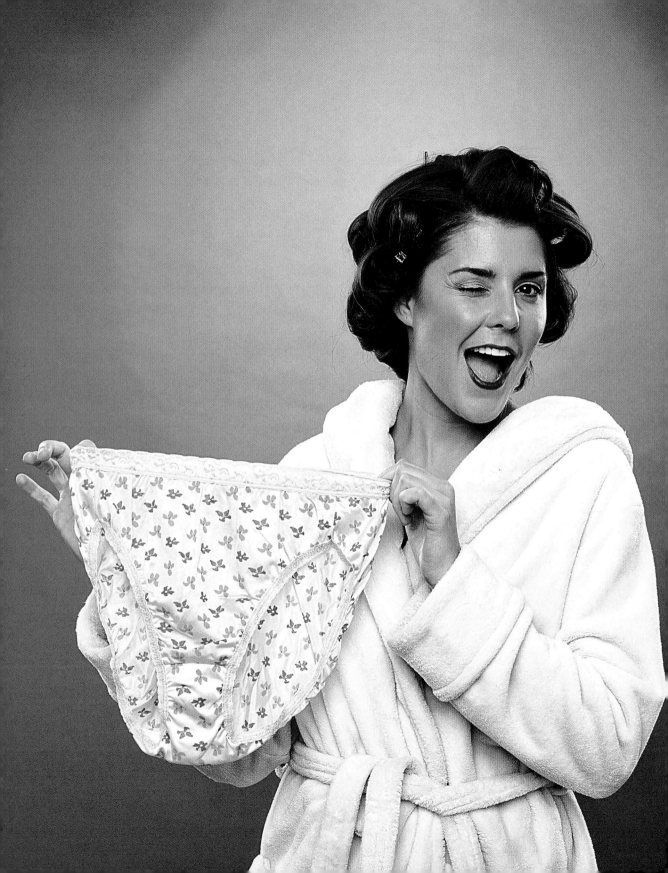

HOW TO

GET READY FOR/ GO ON A DATE

OMG! YOU'RE GOING ON A DATE! OMGOMGOMG! What do you wear? What do you shave? What do your feet smell like? Wait, is that smell your feet or your cooter?

There's a lot to think about! It can be a very stressful experience. I, personally, love dates . . . and equally hate dates. They're fun when they go well and just plain awful when they don't.

One of the most memorable dates I've ever had was with my first college boyfriend. We met on the indoor track team. At one point in my college career, I thought it'd be NEAT to do sports.

I instantly learned it was not. It was a waste of my time, and also I was not as good at track as I thought I was in high school. The only thing I got out of it was a lousy boyfriend.

Except he wasn't lousy, he was very nice and tall and had pretty blue eyes and was decently fast for an upper-middle-class white boy. We had gotten together over winter break and went on a few pseudo-dates; for example, we went to the McDonald's drive-through and ordered Happy Meals (BECAUSE WE WERE SO QUIRKY AND FUN) and we went to Boston Market a few times, too.

But on Valentine's Day we had our first REAL date. I think it was the first date-date I had ever been on. Every other time I'd hung out with a guy, it was in a group situation or supes caz (that's kid talk for "super casual"). This was the first time a guy I was with had MADE A RESERVATION. WTF? THIS IS CLASSY.

And it wasn't just any reservation; it was a reservation to MACARONI GRILL. The classiest of all the chain restaurants! If you've never been to a Macaroni Grill, it's a lovely Italian dining experience in which you can color on the paper tablecloths. CLASSY.

I immediately went to the mall and bought the shortest, yet still sophisticated, black-and-white skirt I could find. It had a metal chain draped on the side for decoration—I felt like the prettiest little Avril Lavigne knockoff. Valentine's Day came and my boyfriend picked me up from my dorm and said, "Whoa, you look hot." He had a way with words. I felt like a South Jersey Cinderella.

He took me to Macaroni Grill and it was hot and crowded and the waiters were in the weeds and sweaty and flustered and not that nice and I loved it. We talked and colored, and colored some more to distract ourselves from the fact that we didn't have a lot to talk about.

After dinner, we went back to his dorm and drank Smirnoff Ice and I gave him his V-Day gift: my virginity. I was so hopped up on the classiness of the dinner-reservation experience that I thought, *TONIGHT'S THE NIGHT.*

Over the course of the two years that we dated, my boyfriend and I went to Macaroni Grill approximately zero more times. Young love.

See, dates can be great! But also don't forget that they can be terrible. So, let me give you my quick tips for both preparing for and going on a date.

Absolute

Be ABSOLUTELY clear that this is, in fact, a date.

When one person doesn't know that it's a date, it can get awkward. Fast. Ack.

It's like ordering a pizza and your friend thinks you said you were ordering shoes and when the pizza comes, he puts it on his feet and you're all like, "Da fuq, Greg?"

Don't be afraid to ask. It's better to find out in advance than to wear your shortest black-and-white JCPenney skirt only to discover when the appetizers come that your "date" wants to talk to you about how you could work together. Professionally. Not in terms of puzzling together sweaty crevices. EEP.

(re)Search

Do your research.

Google them. Lord knows they're going to Google you, if they haven't already. I'm not saying you should download their entire life history like you're on some sort of CIA mission. Just poke around to get a general sense of your date. Make sure he's not a serial killer—unless you're into that kind of thing.

When making conversation, it's helpful to know what your date might be interested in discussing.

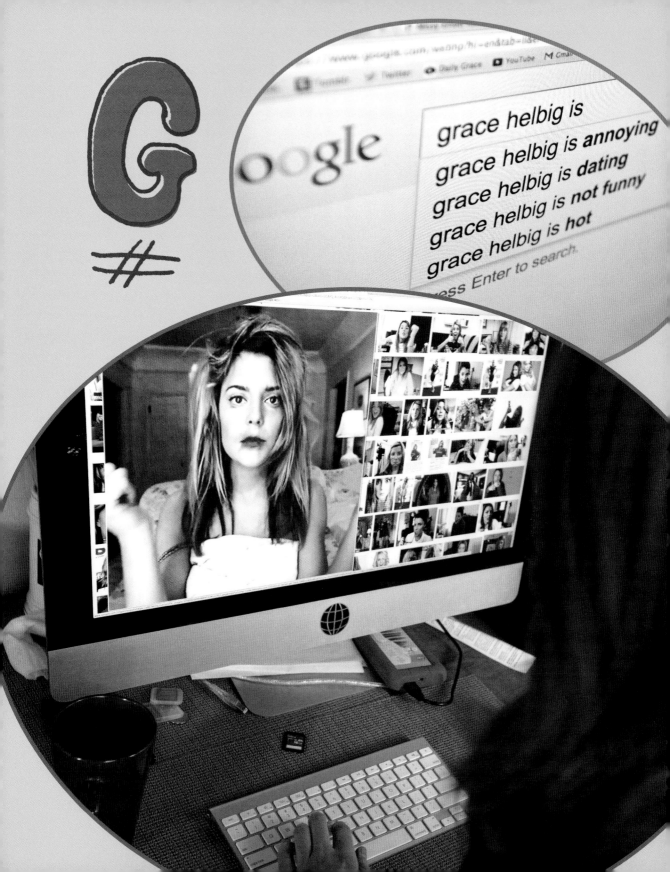

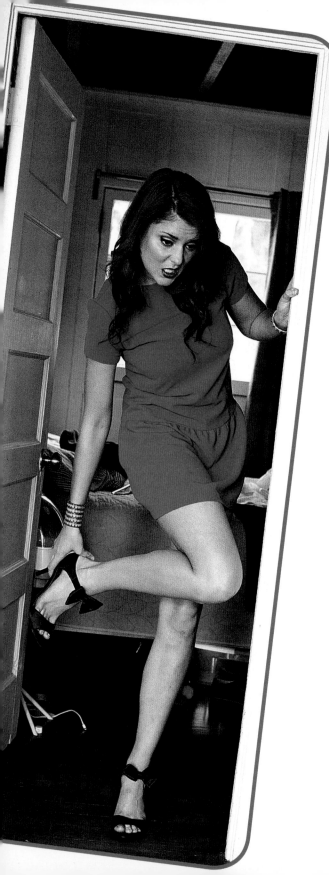

Maybe, when you're researching, you discover that you have some common interests.

Or maybe you fall into the K-hole that is their Facebook photos and spend hours dissecting what kind of girls/boys they've dated in the past.

Maybe you accidentally type their name as your Facebook status. ABORT MISSION.

Whatever you do, don't mention during the date that you Googled the other person. It sounds creepy out loud.

Scrub Up

Clean your person!

Get into the crevices. Have hair only in the places you want it. Use Q-tips! Present the best possible version of yourself. Unless, you're like, *Screw it, I'm kind of gross and I want them to like me for me*. Then you do you. (And hopefully them. HEYO!)

Present the version of yourself that you'd want to date.

Exit Strategy

Figure out an exit strategy, in case of emergencies.

If your love interest turns out to be truly, horribly uninteresting or if they stink emotionally and physically and you just can't stand another minute with this person or you're going to stab your own eyeballs, you should have a way to get out of the date before you get stuck. Whether it's having a friend on standby to send you a "your dog is puking out the butt" text or a cohort at the actual bar/restaurant/café to make sure your date isn't there to wear your skin (can you tell I'm a paranoid human being? Thanks, local news!), or even just a few preloaded "excuses," taking one of these precautionary measures will help you make a break for it if things get weird.

I hate calling them excuses—I prefer WPBBOFTS (We're Probably Both Better Off for This Stories). Fun and creative! It sounds sucky, but the truth is, if you're not having a genuinely fun time, then neither will your date. So it's better to cut your losses and get out of there.

Yes

Say "Yes" to this experience. Stay positive about the date.

What I mean by "Yes" is keep an open mind, especially if you're on the fence about the date. Have an emergency exit plan, but stay on the date until there's truly no better option than to pull the rip cord.

If my foreign language studies have served me correctly, I'm pretty sure "date" comes from the Latin root *date*, which means "awkward situation." Yes, dates are inherently awkward, so give it a chance. Give it the ole two-thirds try. Get through at least two-thirds of the date before you give up. And who knows, maybe by the time you get to the two-thirds point there'll be enough forward momentum to push you through to the end.

And if you're still wearing your own skin at the end of the date, consider it a complete success!

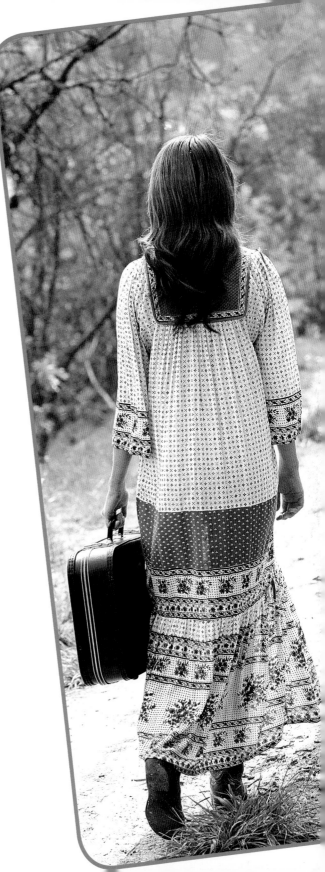

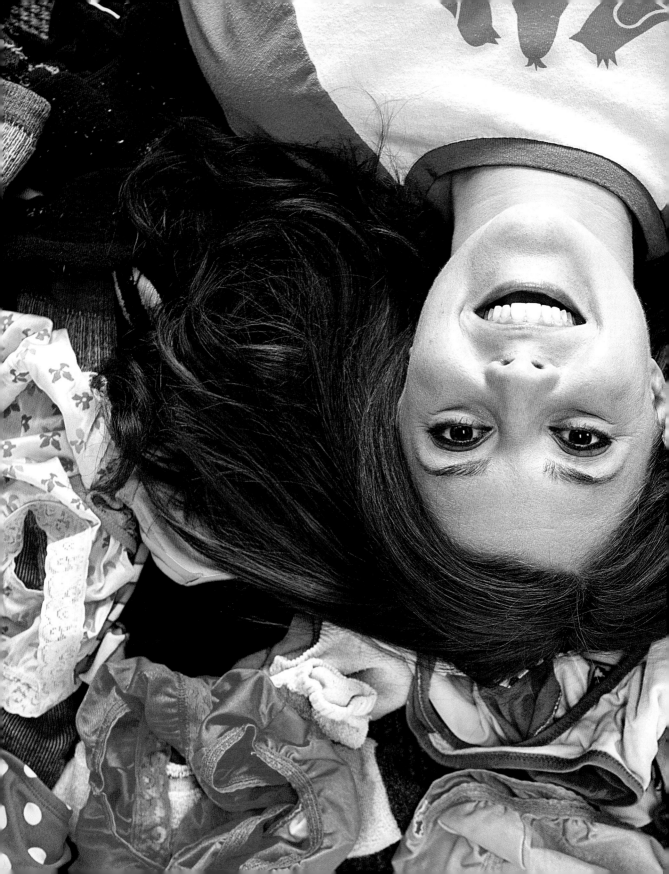

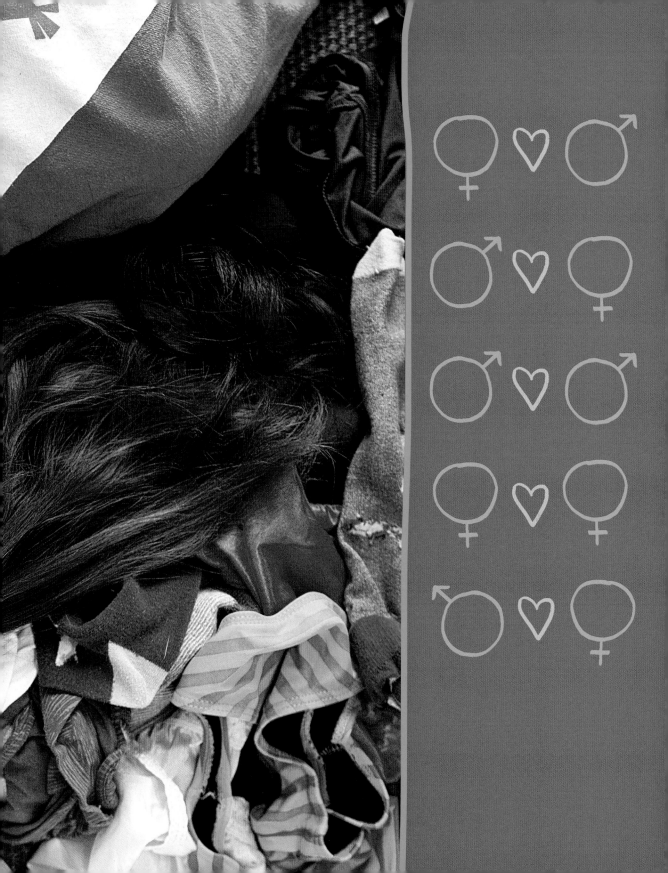

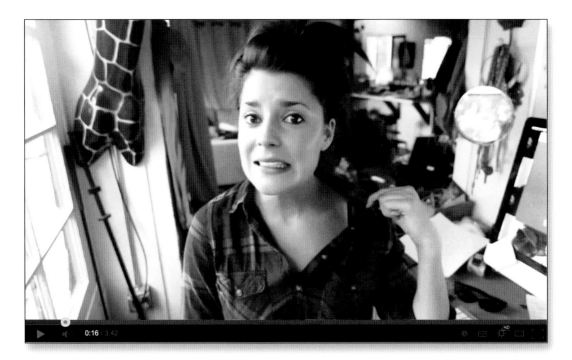

0:16 / 3:42

Dependable

Be dependable. Be on time.

I'm what some might refer to as a "putzer." I waste all the available prep time until I'm late. I have a latent fear of arriving somewhere first, because then I'd have to sit alone and thus feel wildly vulnerable and/or bad about myself. Some might say it can be attributed to deep-seated friendship breakup issues from high school. "Some" would be therapists. HOW FUN. I'm dealing with it. But this is about you! How dare you turn this on me, me.

This is the first impression you'll give your date. Also, side note, it's kind of nice to get to the bar early and order a drink before your date gets there so you don't have to go through the whole

"Oh, what are you drinking? That sounds nice [gag], maybe I'll try that" shenanigans. You have a few minutes to get yourself settled, so your date sees you in the best light. Dim bar lighting is very flattering!

Ask Questions

This is a general rule of thumb for any social situation.

It's something I learned from my dad (I don't have daddy issues [that I know about], you pervs). My dad used to call my brothers and me every night to say, "Wazzzz up." But we were young and quiet, so my dad used to engage us in conversation by asking us question after question about our days/lives. And slowly, as I grew older,

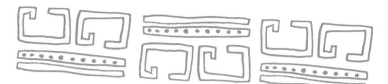

I adopted this method of communicating with people. Always fun to associate your dad with your dating strategies! But, goddamn it, it's very effective.

People who love to talk about themselves love a good "question-asker." And if your date is interested in learning more about you, too, they'll usually toss the question(s) back at you.

Not only is asking questions a great way to keep conversation going, but it's also a great way to spot incredibly egocentric personalities who aren't interested in your thoughts/fears/life and will never ask you any questions in return. Avoid these people.

Decide

Decide how you'd like the date to end.

This will (hopefully) alleviate some of the awkwardness inherent in the end-of-date good-bye.

Do you want to kiss this person? Do you think they'll want to kiss you? Is it a cheek kiss? A closed-mouth, full-lip kiss? An open-mouth lip kiss? An open-mouth, minimal-tongue kiss? Or an open-mouth, maximum-tongue kiss? Is it a handshake? Is it a handshake with the other hand gently touching the top of the shake? Is it a handshake pulled into a hug? Is it a side hug? A full-arms hug? Are both arms up, or both down? Or one arm up and one down? A full-arms, pelvis-away hug? A full-arms, pelvis-in hug? A full-arms, pelvis-out, back-pat hug? A full-arms, pelvis-in, back-rub hug? Is it a no-touch casual wave? Is it a high-five?

There are a lot of options. Figure out what you think is best for the situation. The "good-bye dance" of two bodies not fully committing to hug vs. shake vs. cheek kiss vs. arm placement is not a fun dance. It's why they never do that dance at weddings. The electric slide is way more fun.

And trust me, I need to practice what I preach. I'm awful at committing to a good-bye maneuver.

If things go awry, try to embrace the awkwardness . . . along with the other person's body. Things can only get less awkward from here! And you'll both have a "thing" that you can joke about on future dates. Oh, classic, you guys.

Plain

Order plain food. This is not the time to be an adventurous eater.

Maybe this is just a personal problem, but my stomach is a wild, unpredictable beast machine. I should probably see a doctor. Remind me at the end of this book to make an appointment. Thanks, reader friend!

My stomach gets even worse when I'm in any relatively stressful situation. So I highly, HIGHLY recommend that if you're on a date in which consuming food is part of the activity, opt for things that are plain and simple and won't cause any digestive confrontations. You know your body better than anyone (outside of your gynecologist), so you know what will confuse and what will amuse your intestines.

Life tip: Don't be on the outs with your intestines. Especially when you're trying to make a good first impression.

Let your personality be explosive, not your butthole.

Original

Be original.

Don't let your anxiety about the date make you boring. Uh-oh, here comes some after-school-special tough love. Remember to be yourself, dummy! Cue the rainbow-and-stars graphic with the tagline "The More You Don't Blow."

This might seem like hollow beauty pageant advice, but it's good to be reminded. Same goes for life in general—have your own opinions, emotions, thoughts, and overall point of view. Make sure your date isn't out to dinner with a sheep. Because that's illegal.

Pregnant

Try not to get pregnant on the first date.

Or the second, really. There are a variety of ways to prevent this, but I will let you research those on your own. Best of luck.

And there you go. You did it! You got ready for and went on a date. Hopefully, it wasn't the worst experience of your whole life. But if it was, things can only get better from here, so congrats on hitting rock bottom!

Side note joke: If Dwayne Johnson was a drag queen, his name would be Rock Bottom.

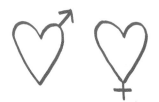

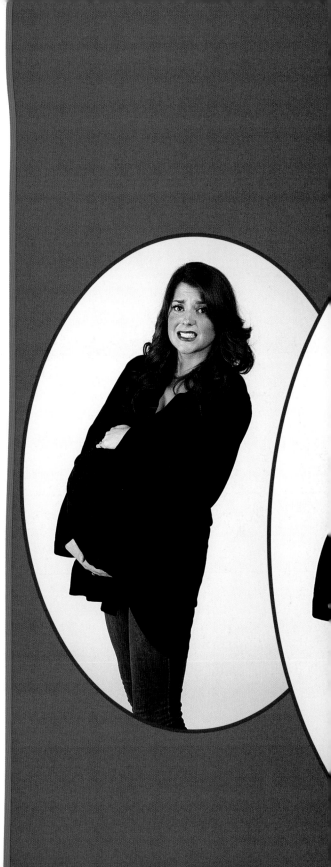

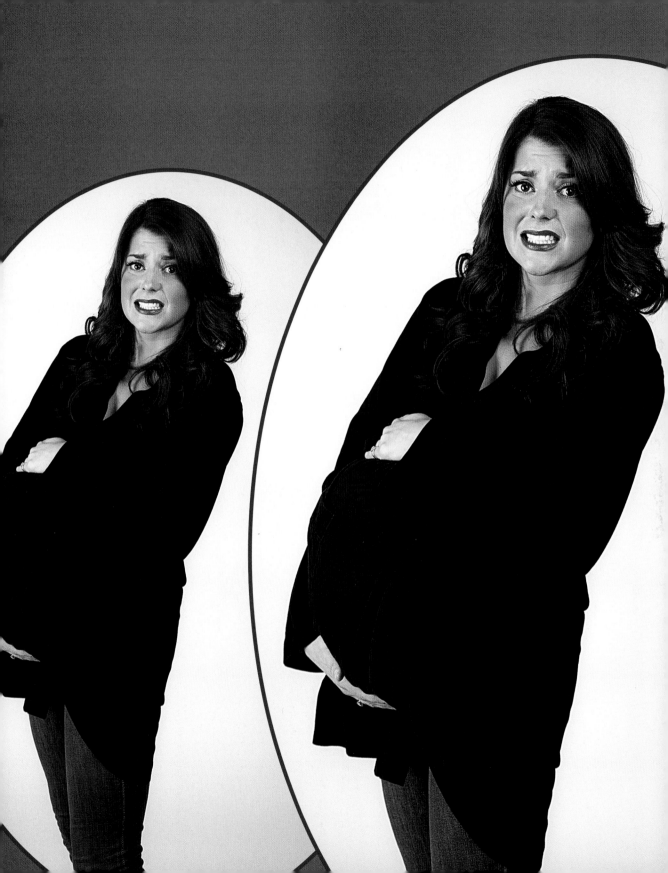

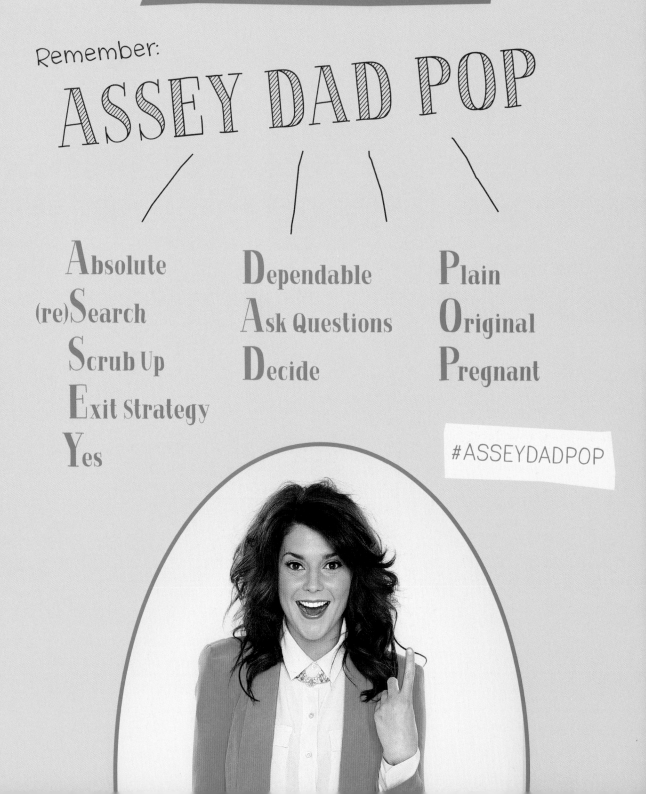

□ CHECKLIST □

THINGS TO BRING ON A DATE

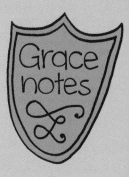

☐ **1.** **ID.** If you get roofied, you'll want people to be able to identify you.

☐ **2.** **Cell phone (fully charged).** It can be used to text friends to get you out of there/as a mirror for food-in-teeth situations/overall friend if you get stood up.

☐ **3.** **Tampons.** Just always have these with you, especially if you're one of those "adventurous types" who wears white pants (god bless).

☐ **4.** **Lipstick.** This can double as blush! How quaint! Or as fake blood if you really need to fake an emergency.

☐ **5.** **Money/payment options.** You're not a damsel in distress, you're a damsel in dis dress THAT YOU PAID FOR (but if they really want to pay, just let them, don't make it weird).

☐ **6.** **Mouth-freshening devices.** It's gross to kiss someone who tastes like Alfredo sauce.

☐ **7.** **Meds.** For weird stomachs/anxiety/headaches/whatever your body system might scream for.

☐ **8.** **Backup underwear.** This sounds scandalous, but you NEVER KNOW, so always be prepared.

☐ **9.** **Deodorant.** Bring this everywhere all the time.

☐ **10.** **Confidence.** Or at least a false sense of it.

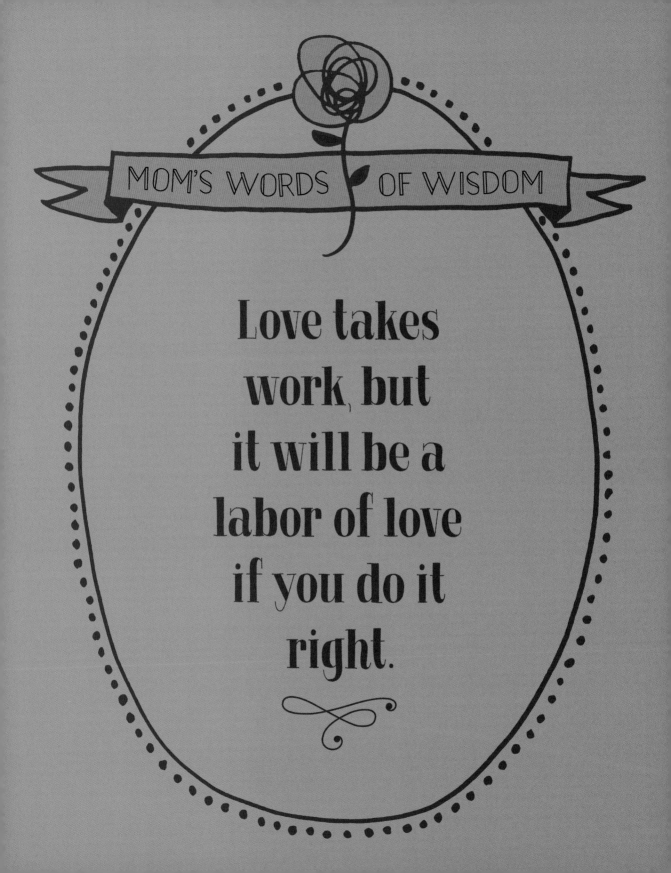

MOM'S WORDS OF WISDOM

Love takes
work, but
it will be a
labor of love
if you do it
right.

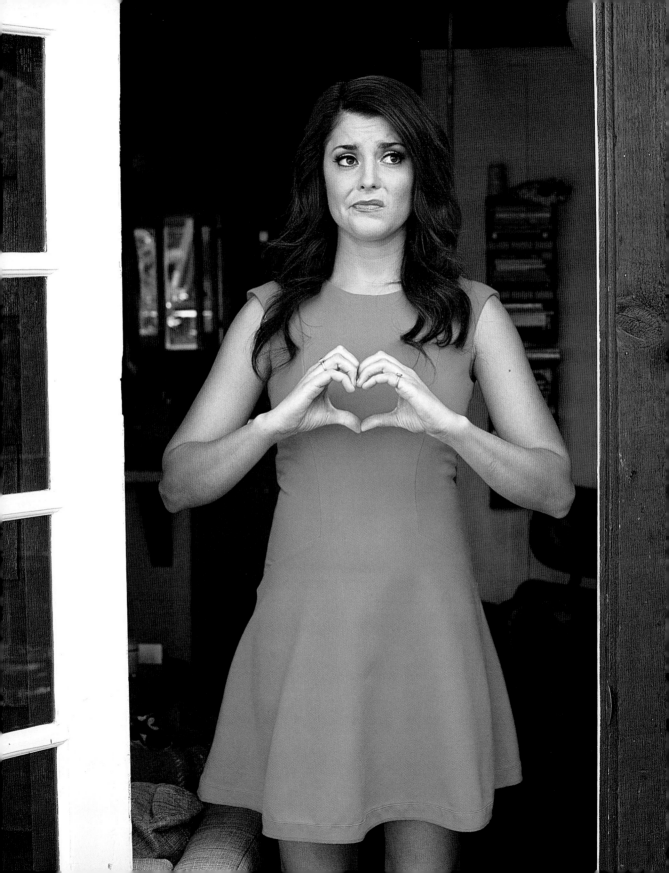

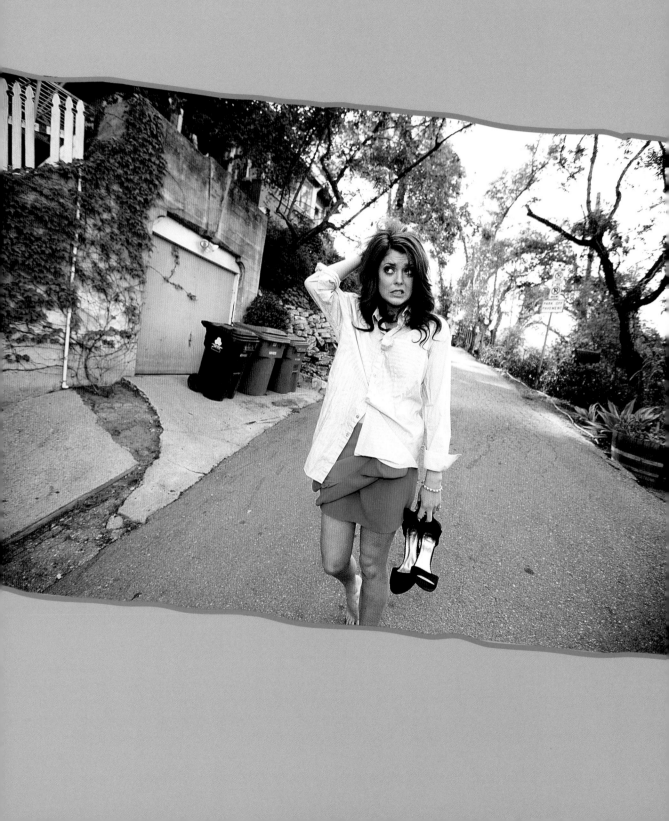

HOW TO

DO THE WALK OF SHAME

Oh, the walk of shame. It happens to the best of us. A wonderful emotional and physical journey from "What" to "Oh" to "Uh-oh" to "God-damn it" to a plume of smoke left behind after you run out the door. WOSs aren't just for the ladies. They're like STDs—they're for everyone!

I've done a few WOSs in my day and, optimistically speaking, I feel that they've made me a more resourceful, inventive, and capable person. They teach you to think on your feet, because lord knows you were thinking on your back last night. HEYO!

Here's a quick list of some things that may or may not have happened to me before, during, or after WOSs.

- Greeted my neighbors barefoot, with smeared eyeliner (while they had a baby in a stroller—even that baby knew).
- Surrendered my underwear to a stranger's apartment floor.
- Left a REALLY GREAT leather jacket that I finally convinced myself to buy because I was "investing in myself"—turns out I lied to myself.
- Dry-heaved in a park.
- Silently convinced myself that my "look" was "hipster" and "purposeful."
- Locked myself out of my apartment.
- Had someone drive me home in a pickup truck (that was more of a ride of shame).
- Ran into a notable college professor.

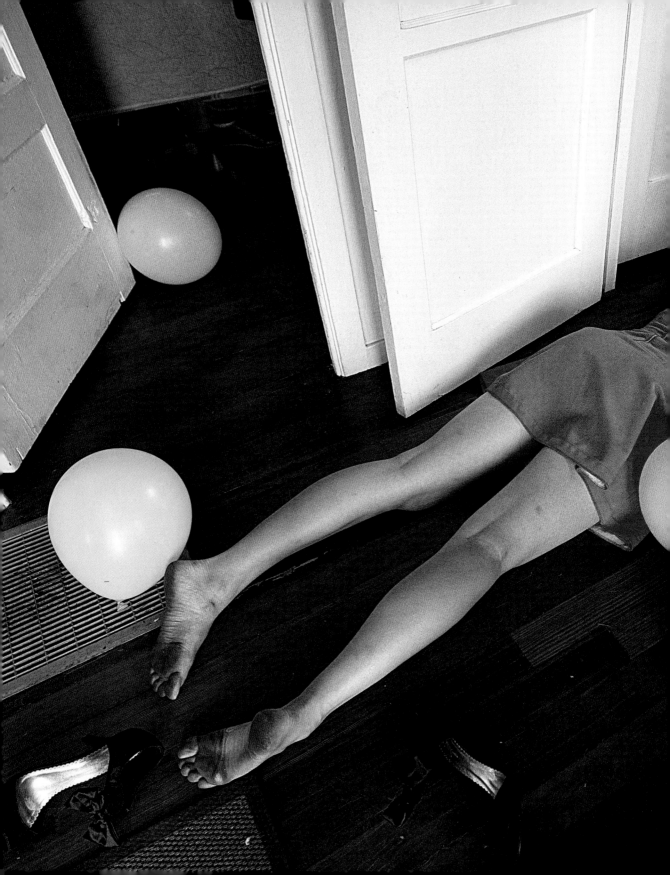

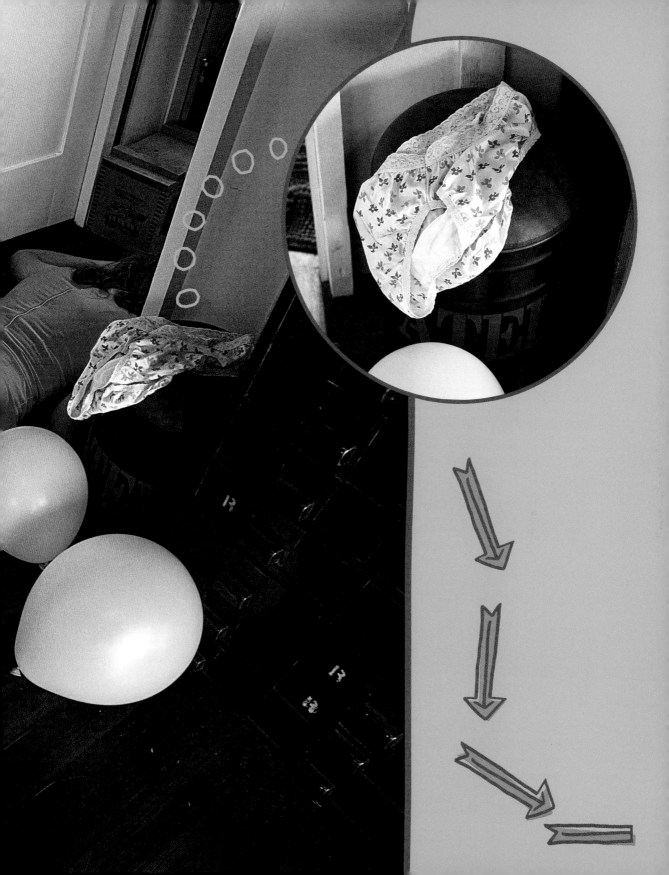

- Fell asleep on the subway and ended up in Coney Island.
- Forgot that I accidentally lit part of my hair on fire the night before and thought I slept with a scientist that poured chemicals on me in the middle of the night.
- Consoled myself with SO much bacon.

WOSs teach us a lot about ourselves. Our strengths. Our weaknesses. Our questionable taste in human company at two a.m. They teach us that scrubbing your skin in the shower for an hour doesn't erase the memories. They teach us that no amount of Bath & Body Works Cashmere Glow body splash can cover up a sexual blooper. They teach us that calling it a sexual blooper makes it sound less like a mistake and more like a silly accident you won't repeat. Hopefully. But c'est la pee(nis) (peh heh heh, NAILED IT).

Here are my tips and tricks for turning the walk of shame into a walk of fame. But we all know you had enough tips and tricks last night. Dick tips and sex tricks . . . I'll go.

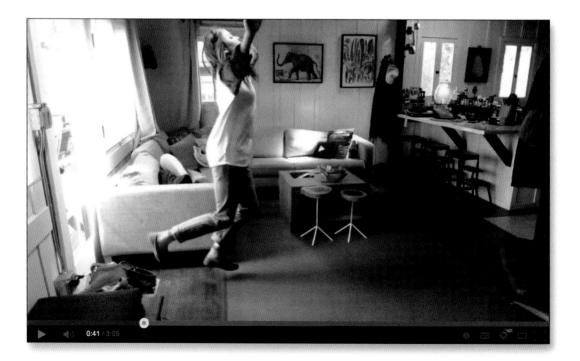

Sike, I'm back. But for you there's no going back, so let's get you out of there!

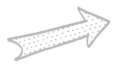
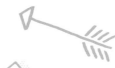

Where

Where are you?

That's the first question you should ask. Are you familiar with this place? Who's next to you? Who's on the couch? Who's on the floor in the bathroom? What country are you in? Where's your car?

No matter where you are, the only question that really matters is: How do I get home from here?

Accept

Accept that this has happened.

It might take a few seconds or minutes, but resign yourself to the fact that this is, in fact, happening right now.

It's best not to waste your time being angry or upset or disappointed. Save those feelings for the super-long shower you will definitely take later. Now's the time to focus on the process of getting your person and possessions out of here.

Find

Find your things.

Remember that all you really need in order not to be considered a complete and utter wreck are: your wallet (with ID and credit cards), phone, keys, and some kind of clothing. Anything else you recover is a bonus.

Think of this part like it's a video game where you have to find treasures in an uncharted land (you'll notice that my knowledge of video games

is both vast and accurate). This should help make the search for your underwear seem fun instead of humiliating. Bonus points when you locate your bra and panties! Go team!

Remember, if you can't find your own clothes, there are a lot of things around you that could be made into clothing/genital coverings of some sort. More bonus points!

Never feel bad about stealing clothes. Truly, you've earned them. Wear them like a purple heart and then burn them when you get home.

Exits

Locate the exits!

Imagine you're on a plane and one of the flight attendants is giving the spiel about locating the closest exits in the event of an emergency, and you're like, *Blah blah blah. OHHHH, let's see what kind of food they offer on this flight. Do I want a Bloody Mary or a vodka soda? Whoa, ham and cheese on a CROISSANT? Delta, you fancy.*

Well, the time has finally come to locate your nearest exit. This is an emergency.

Figure out the best route to the door that is the least likely to wake anyone up or cause you to accidentally stumble into someone else's room or possibly interact with a stranger. Get to the outside. Escape out a window if you have to.

Resist

Resist the urge to say good-bye.

This will only complicate things. You don't owe the other person a good-bye or an explanation

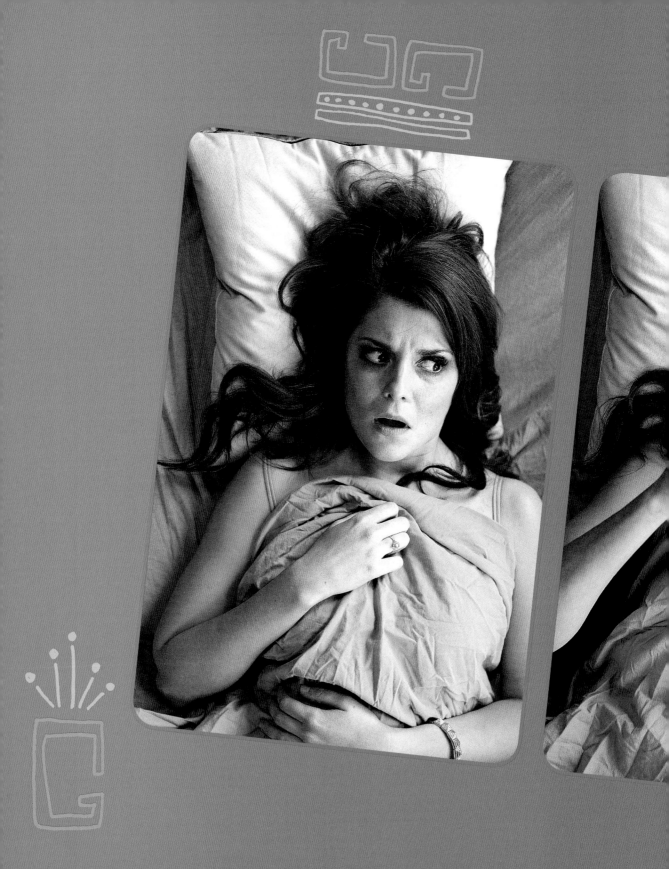

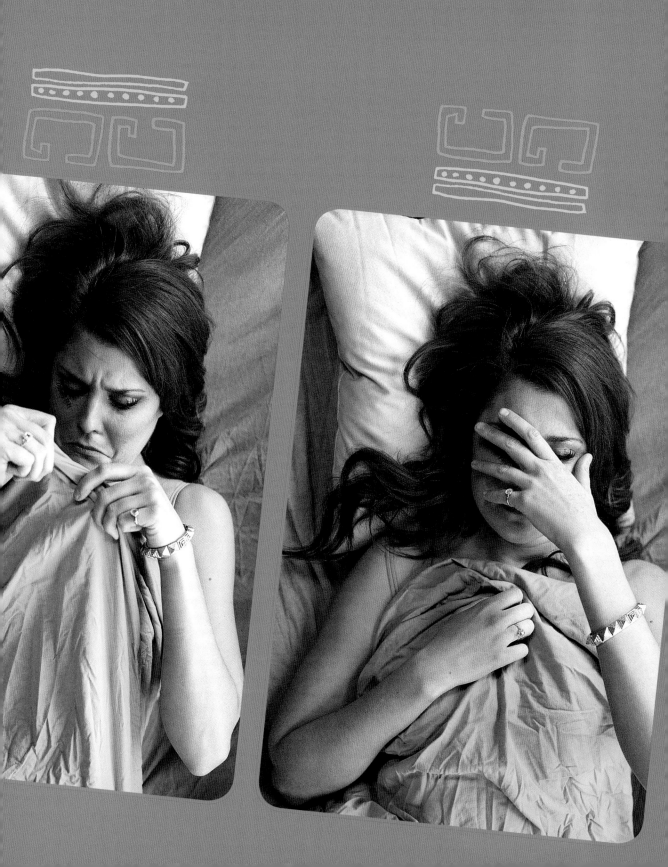

for why you're leaving. And who knows, maybe a conversation isn't exactly what they want, either. You're doing everyone a favor. This is an Irish Good-bye.

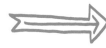

Texts

If you have a second, check your text messages.

Make a quick scan of your social media. This step is not completely necessary and can be saved for after you've left. It might help you start to piece together things from last night and help you craft the story you'll be telling people about what happened (a step that'll come later).

The next morning, I can always tell if I've had a bonkers night by checking my photos. When I reach a crazy-town level of intoxication, I become convinced that I'm an amazing photographer and start photographing everything. And what I end up with are a series of dark, out-of-focus blurs, with one (maybe) relatively decipherable image that hints at the subject I was trying so desperately to capture.

An **Irish Good-bye** is when you leave a party or social situation without saying good-bye to anyone. Typically, this happens because you're too "crunk" on the "sizzyrup." Whatever your nationality is, it doesn't matter, because today you're Irish. And it's fitting, because you probably drank like you were Irish last night.

I'll also find terrible bathroom mirror selfies. I take a lot of those when I'm hurting my liver. I'm a true artist.

Check to see whom you've contacted, or who's contacted you. Did you tweet or post anything incriminating? Did anyone else? Did your annoying friend Meg text you, "where are u???" "r u ok??" "brunch?!" You don't have to reply right now; it's just helpful to know whom you'll have to explain things to later.

Ass

Do you smell like it?

There's a chance you'll run into other functioning members of society once you've escaped your current situation. I like to carry travel-sized deodorants with me in my bags and car. Not because I engage in WOSs on the regular, but because I regularly forget to put on deodorant in my normal life.

If you can't locate any deodorant, there are a lot of things that can mask an odor. Or at least sort of mask it. Half mask it. Like the Phantom

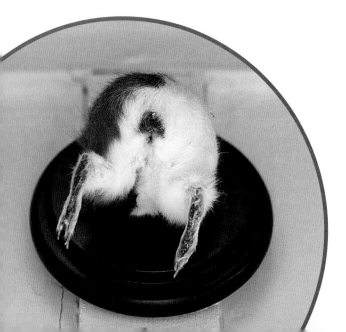

of the Opera. For instance, soap. You don't have to wash yourself (unless you really want to take a shower in a stranger's bathroom, or you have some sort of OCD thing and you have to), but if you rub soap on your wrists and neck it can help! At least I tell myself that.

Other things you can rub on yourself to create a more pleasant odor include, but are not limited to, candles, dish soap, any body splash, mouthwash, Lysol, air fresheners, magazine perfume samples, and scented markers.

Be creative, you can find something. Or just be prepared to run all the way home.

Invent

Invent the story you'll tell everyone.

You'll need to step it up and become a professional, inventive narrator, because odds are the true story of what happened last night isn't that great.

Unless it's great. Then tell that story. Be proud of your mistakes. Mistakes are what allow us to learn and grow or something. Right. I defer to Deepak Chopra on this one.

But this is my book, so let's make some stuff up! Remember to keep the story airtight. Don't allow your friends to find holes. This isn't *Memento*. Even though you are remembering things backward. So it's kind of *Memento*.

Keep it simple. It'll be easier to remember.

Also, keep it consistent. Tell the same story. It might slowly become the truth in your mind and help you forget what really happened. Yay!

 ow

Now, get out!

You've probably already spent more time here than you should have, so skedaddle.

Possible stories

- You ran into a troll under a bridge and you both decided to do a half marathon.
- You were visiting your local art museum and there was an interactive art exhibit about interpretive dance.
- You got dragged into a late-night church contact dodgeball game.
- You found a stray dog and took it to a twenty-four-hour vet and then its owner came by and reclaimed it only after you engaged in a heated argument about their neglect.
- You were up all night donating to charity.
- You left the bar and decided that tonight's the night you finally respond to your pen pal.
- A skunk sprayed you.
- You followed someone you thought was Leonardo DiCaprio for hours before you realized it was Michael Fassbender—d'oh!
- You spent your night scratching lottery tickets with a talking cat.

Did you leave yet?
LEAVE.
GO.
GET TO THE OUTSIDE.

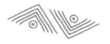

Take

Oh, but before you go, feel free to take something.

I'm not saying take money out of a wallet. You're not a prostitute. Unless you are, then you shouldn't be reading this. For you, this isn't a walk of shame, this is a job.

Take some food, or a beverage, or some gum, or a shirt, or a light fixture that's super cute. The possibility of you ever seeing this person again in real life is inversely related to the retail value of the object you take. The less likely you are to see them again, the nicer the thing you can take. Smiley face emoticon.

And there you have it. Now scurry back to your own cave via whatever is the easiest, fastest, most private route you can manage.

As embarrassing or regretful as this experience may have been, it's helpful to remember that you ended the night at their place, not yours. And that was a pro move.

It's so much easier to escape the situation when you're at someone else's place than it is to wake up with a random person in your own bed. If that happens to you, maybe try locking yourself in the bathroom until they leave. But that's a chapter for a whole other time. Not that you'll be reading it later in this book, because I didn't write that chapter. Should I have written that chapter? Nah. I CAN'T DO EVERYTHING FOR YOU GUYS.

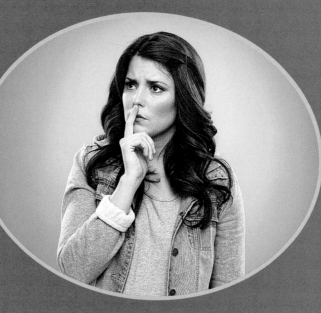

Remember:

WAFER TAINT

Where	Texts
Accept	Ass
Find	Invent
Exits	Now
Resist	Take

#WAFERTAINT

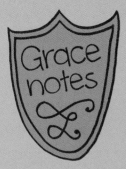

□ MAD LIBS □

WALK OF SHAME

Here's what happened: It was a regular night out at my favorite bar, _____.
[name of bar]

you know, the place that had that _____ scare that one time? That place.
[animal]

But right when I was about to get my _____ and my _____, my
[food]   [food]

classic order, I was abducted by _____ and taken to _____,
[plural noun]   [city/country/planet]

where I was _____. The worst part of it was that they drove
[verb past tense]

a _____. Hello, it's not _____! Inside the _____, I met the leader of
[vehicle]   [year]   [type of building]

the _____, _____. But everyone called _____ _____.
[plural noun]   [name]   [he/she/it]   [nickname]

_____ was very _____ and I couldn't help but _____ at
[he/she/it]   [adjective]   [verb]

_____ _____ because it smelled like _____. Also _____
[his/her/its] [body part]   [adjective]   [he/she/it]

had a very visible tramp stamp of a _____. _____. _____ gave
[tattoo]   [adjective]   [he/she/it]

me a specific _____ and told me I must protect it or risk my _____.
[noun]   [noun]

They clearly don't know about how I lost _____'s _____. Woof.
[name]   [noun]

But just when I thought they were going to _____ me, _____ ran
[verb]   [name]

into the room and _____ me. We _____ all the way back
[verb past tense]   [verb past tense]

to _____ until we found a _____ diner named _____ and
[city/state/planet]   [adjective]   [noun]

had _____ _____ shots. I don't remember much else
[number]   [adjective + animal name]

about the night, but I owe my _____ to _____ and my virginity.
[noun]   [name]

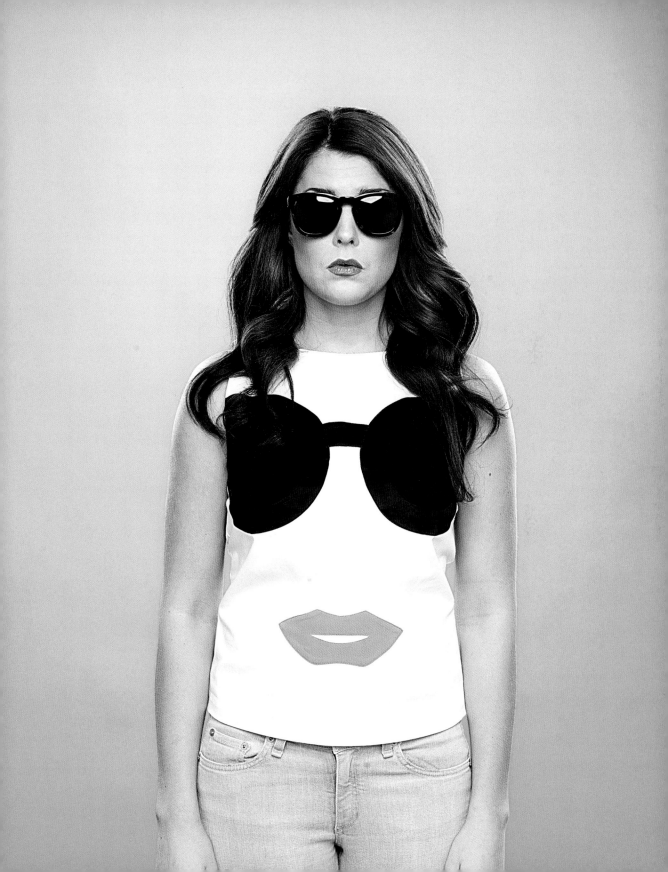

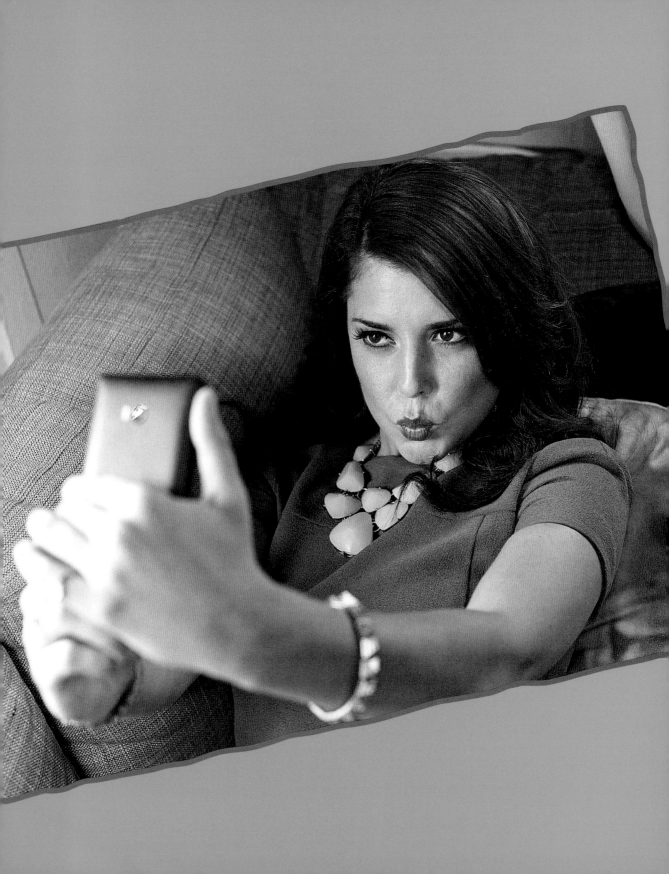

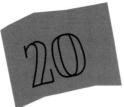

DIGITAL DATING TIPS

In just a few years, the Internet has managed to boil down the age-old tradition of matchmaking to a finger swipe. A finger swipe. Swipe one way or "like" a future potential love interest's profile, and you might be one step closer to finding love (or a booty call). And if you happen to mis-swipe you could miss your soul mate. What a treat!

The standard rule of thumb for Internet dating is: things may not be exactly as they seem. Objects in the rearview mirror may appear closer than they are. Even though I've never noticed that. Have you? To me they always seem like they're at the accurate distance from the mirror. Then again, I have terrible spatial awareness. My legs and arms are constantly bruised from bumping into things on a daily basis. But enough about me, let's talk more about me.

I created a profile on OkCupid once. It was for a video. I dressed up like Justin Bieber and took a photo and created a profile under the pseudonym Dale Burndart. I filled out next to nothing in the profile, except that I was thirty-five, male, and lived in Brooklyn.

My photo was blurry and unflattering and overall just completely dumb. But to this day, I still get alerts from OkCupid that there are interested ladies who want to communicate with me. I don't know what's worse—that these women are looking for love in the wrong place or that my picture so easily tricked them into thinking I was a man. Look, I've inherited a lot of my dad's features. I'm cool with it. My passport photo looks like it belongs to a European male tennis player.

Digital dating can be daunting, so here are twenty quick tips that might help.

1. **Ask a friend or two whom you trust and respect to look at your profile.** Have them describe it to you in three quick words or phrases without hesitation. Is their description in line with what you're trying to project to the cyber universe? If not, there's room for improvement. In a way, you're selling yourself, so make sure your profile is "on brand" and true to you. Babies "R" Us doesn't sell dildos. This is a terrible example.

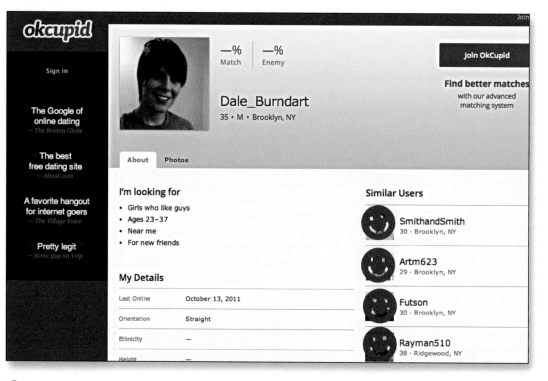

2. If the person you're pursuing online uses "LOL" unironically more than once either in their profile or in any conversational exchange, you should GTFO. I can guarantee you they're not laughing out loud, and if they are, then they're too generous with their laughter. Someone hurt them at some point in their lives. They have baggage. Keep moving.

3. If they have "I love the beach" in their profiles, shut it down. You're about to engage with a generic human Hallmark card. Unless they're telling you they like the beach because they have an abnormal deep-seated lust and sexual desire for the beach and are looking for someone else who's on their unique psychological level, then yes, they should have that in their profile.

4. If you want someone to respond to you, try ending your message with a question. This seems so extremely obvious, but it's easy to get caught up in the excitement of online interaction and just send a message quickly that doesn't completely set you up for success with a reply.

5. Beware of shirtless and/or bikini profile photos. These intentionally sexy photos may cause you to overlook other important qualities in a potential mate. Remember, bodies get gross over time but the brain is forever-ish.

6. Could you imagine yourself pooping in the room next to them? This really only applies to you if you're looking for a serious relationship. Relationships are about making yourself vulnerable. And one of the most vulnerable acts is #2-ing in the same vicinity as someone you want to swap body spit with later. Yes, it's something you'll both probably try to avoid in the beginning, but the body can only hold out for so

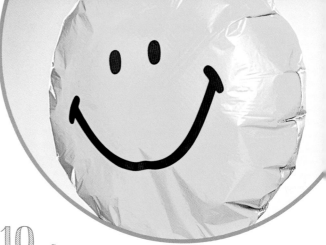

long and once you both cross the threshold your bond will deepen. This might sound like a crazy tip, but I truly believe in it.

7. Use emoji sparingly. Dating shouldn't have to be a rebus. (Google it, I definitely did.) Sure, they're fun and stupid, but at the end of the day you're an adult, use your words. It's cute to date someone who still has a stuffed animal, it's creepy to date someone who still has fifty stuffed animals.

8. If you set up a date that will take place IRL, try meeting in an open, public place. A place where you can't be kidnapped (easily) but could still fake a "business" emergency if it isn't going well and exit the date early without leaving the person awkwardly alone. You're not that coldhearted after all. Good ideas for an IRL date: a park, a decently popular bar for happy hour, a medium-crowded petting zoo. Bad ideas: a hot-air balloon, their old van, a hedge maze.

9. Google yourself to see what comes up. It's helpful to know what's out there about you that a potential future lover might need context or clarity on so they don't get the wrong impression. For instance, I participated in ONE teeny-tiny beauty pageant ONCE six years ago. I didn't even tell my closest friends at the time. But the information got onto the Internet a few years ago and now it's one of the first questions a lot of people ask me about. I was thrown off the first few times it happened, but now I know how to talk about it. And no, I did not win, and yes, I sported a "Jersey pouf" during the evening gown competition. More on this later. Be sure to prep yourself about yourself.

10. Some people are just plain bonk-bonk. (I tried to create a cuter term for "crazy.") Keep away from the bonk.

11. Be cautious about giving out your phone number. Your phone number is like your virginity—a very sacred item. Remember, it's much easier to ignore emails or g-chats than it is to deal with someone regularly texting or calling you.

12. Usually people who have anything about religion in their profiles are more religious than you think. Are you ready to go with God?

13. Group mind! Sometimes it's helpful to work together with friends. I've been out to drinks and have watched one friend use her phone to Google and Facebook a potential match to find out how honest he was being on his profile while another friend had the guy's Tinder profile open and waited with bated fingers. Together we collectively decided he was a "like swipe."

14. FarmersOnly.com is a dating website only for farmers. It's real. This is not a tip so much as a fact. A wonderful fact.

15. Don't let Internet dating become your full-time job. It's a lot of work, but don't let it override your work-work. If it's becoming too much, take a break, go to a bar, observe humans IRL. Once you're sufficiently socially overwhelmed, return to the keyboard.

16. Don't imbibe and Internet. Don't get drunk and peruse the digital meat market. Results may vary. But they're RAREly good.

17. If a guy posts a lot of photos of himself surrounded by girls, it's likely that he's overcompensating for something. He's already trying very hard to prove to you that he's fun and people like him and he's definitely not socially awkward and totally didn't make these strange girls take a photo with him, because he really does know them. Use your judgment. What would Judge Judy say? She's an excellent judge of character.

18. You don't have to go on a second date. There are a lot of people in this world. Don't settle. You're great. THIS IS TOO SINCERE . . . *sneeze-fart sound effect*

19. Be honest. Don't withhold crucial information. If you're five-foot-eight, say you're five-foot-eight. Don't say you're six-foot and show up wearing heeled cowboy boots like they can't tell. It's so much more effort to continuously cover a lie than to try to find a person that likes you for you. And the rewards are so much sweeter. Like a bowl of real Lucky Charms compared to that generic version that tastes like chalk. You know what I'm talking about.

20. All hope is not lost. Keep your chin up. Eventually scientists will make really lifelike pleasure robots and none of us will ever have to worry about dating again!

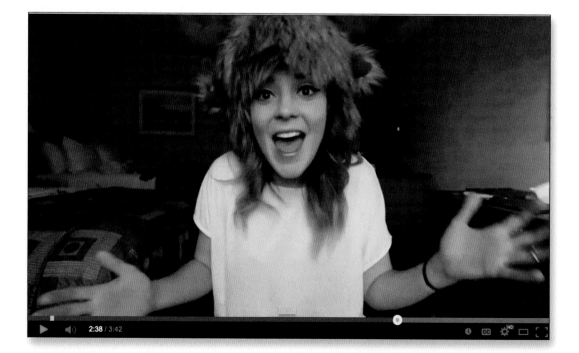

2:38 / 3:42

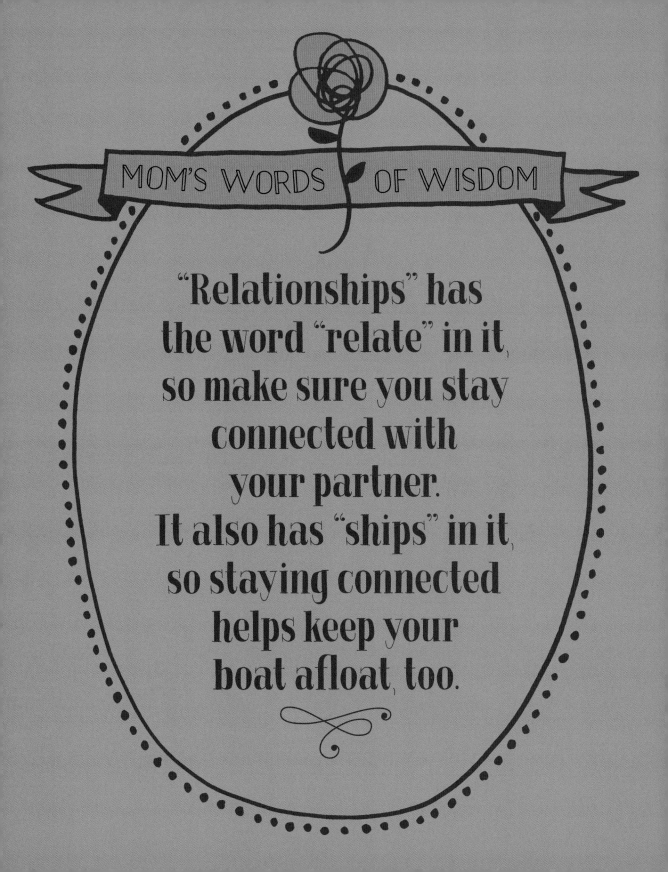

MOM'S WORDS OF WISDOM

"Relationships" has the word "relate" in it, so make sure you stay connected with your partner. It also has "ships" in it, so staying connected helps keep your boat afloat, too.

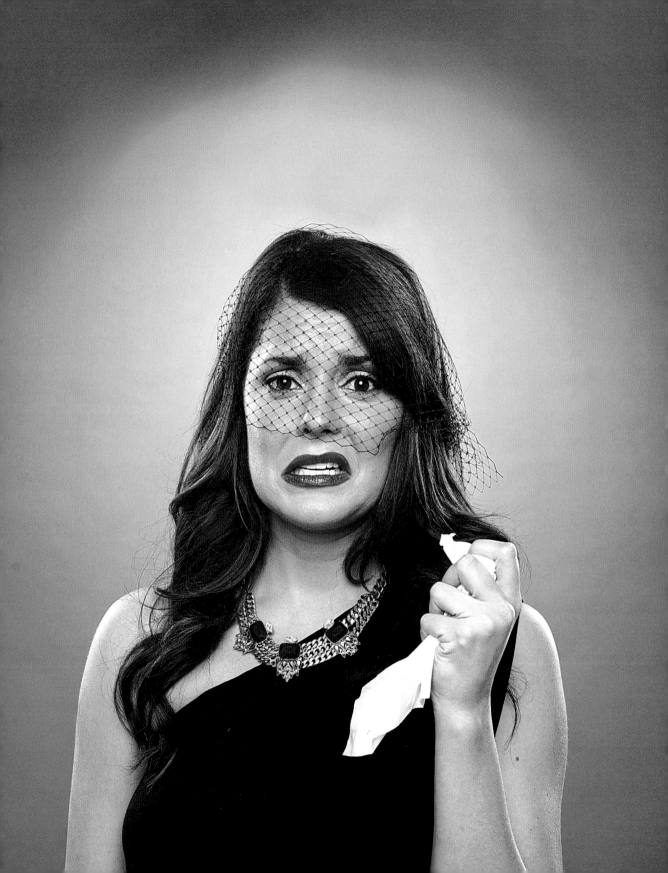

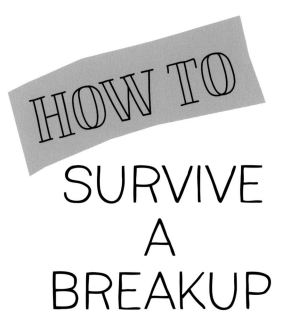

HOW TO SURVIVE A BREAKUP

Breakups suck. Period. No ifs, ands, or buts about it. Well, one less butt about it. SORRY, TOO SOON.

I had the best/worst breakup experience when one of the most meaningful relationships of my life was coming to an end and my boyfriend and I mutually agreed that it was time to move on after three years. We decided to spend a weekend in the famous Chelsea Hotel in Manhattan, so we could let it all out and try to find some closure. We drank and ate and told each other everything we loved and hated about each other and cried and laughed and yelled and sexed and were hungover together. It was wonderful. And then it was done. And we hugged and kissed and left each other on the corner of Twenty-third Street and Sixth Avenue.

Though we had a good breakup, it didn't change the fact that I was devastated. My life became a blur. I was drinking for two—myself and my sadness. I felt pretty numb and barely left my apartment for weeks.

During that time, I got a distinct pleasure out of/released some of my anger by watching the revamped version of the classic TV show *90210*. My roommate and I would yell at the TV about how much we hated it. "ANNIE LEFT THE PROM HUMILIATED AND INSTANTLY RUNS OVER A HOMELESS MAN WITH HER CAR?! REALLY?!!? WHY IS THERE A HOMELESS MAN CROSSING A DESERTED CALIFORNIA MOUNTAIN ROAD?!"

Little by little I tried to get myself more involved in the improv scene and my roommate tried to take me out to his friends' parties. I'll never forget the first time I really laughed and felt something close to joy again. After a late night out with my roommate, we stumbled into our local bodega—the only place still open—desperate for something to eat. It barely had any food stocked, besides a weird variety of canned became a great outlet for me, and when I was ready, I found love again with a cool dude.

You may discover that with time, all of those intense emotions and weird/awkward interactions you had are sort of funny. Looking back, the best/worst part of that breakup weekend was when we went to a nearby Whole Foods to buy "breakup food" (aka anything that could be heated up on our hotel stovetop) and ran into a mutual comedy friend. He asked us what we were doing in that neighborhood and my soon-to-be ex said, "Oh, we're breaking up tonight." Our comedy friend laughed nervously, because he could tell it wasn't a joke.

I waited out the entire interaction in silence. I was both extremely hungover from a night of "relationship analyzing" and completely mortified. Unexpected interactions with other people make me anxious under normal circumstances, let alone during a breakup. Comedy friend and I still sometimes reminisce about the very special awkward time we shared at Whole Foods.

Getting over a breakup is one of those moments when you wish you could freeze time and wallow in your sadness. If that were somehow possible, all personal and professional commitments would magically disappear until you could finish a *Say Yes to the Dress/Dance Moms* marathon. If only.

I know every human in your life is probably overwhelming you with their opinions or some sort of generic "gender power" advice or other words meant to console you but actually don't.

cat foods and black beans. My roommate and I looked at each other and screamed, "BEANS!" in unison, like we hadn't eaten in weeks. We were holding hands, jumping up and down and celebrating, while the guy at the register tried to understand how we functioned on a daily basis. For the next two months I avoided that bodega. But it proved that the dumbest stuff could bring me joy when I least expected it—and I could laugh again.

Over time, I started to feel less depressed and began dating. And eventually I stopped feeling like I was always holding my breath. Comedy

And truth be told, I don't know you. I don't know what you're going through. But I can assume. And you know what happens when you assume? You get ass. Let's do this.

Sad

You're going to be sad.

Try to fight it; I dare you. LET YOURSELF FEEL SAD. Adele makes a lot of money because her songs have a very, very relatable sadness. It's okay to cry.

Angry

You're going to be angry.

This is the point when you realize you can't control the other person's feelings. You can't make them love you. You can't make them like you. You can't make them want to be in the same room with you. You can't make them stop feeling hurt by you. AND THAT SUCKS. Why aren't they our forever-there human robot?

BE PISSED. FEEL IT. Go nuts and let it out. But at the end of the day don't hate yourself. Don't be irrational. Channel your anger into something productive. Like boxing or knitting. Or knitting boxing gloves. Get the toxic energy out of you in whatever way feels right. Write down how you're feeling, but think about whether you really NEED to share your rage with others. Resist doing or saying anything that you'll regret. Your irrational, aggressive, reputation-destroying feelings will pass.

You're classy and cool. You're above all of this. You can be like Kate Middleton! Or at least like the suburban Cayte Myddulton. I believe in you.

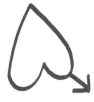

Friends

You need them.

Rely on your friends. This is their moment to shine. Even if you feel like you want to be alone, let them be there.

Your brain is in a fragile state and they'll have a clearer, detached view of what's good and what's bad for you right now. You be the old woman in the nursing home and let them clean out your bedpans. This is a metaphor. If you're using bedpans after a breakup, stop that. And also your friends are too nice.

Eat

Let yourself eat and drink whatever the hell you want.

Cut yourself some slack.

Sleep

Try to.

Sleep might be hard to come by at this time, but do try. God, I sound like your mother, I'm sorry. Unless your mother doesn't care if you sleep. Then I'm sorry you were raised by such a terrible human. I'm here for you. Unless I'm busy. Sorry, I just have a lot of things to do. Get a hobby. Oh wait, hold that thought for a couple pages, that step will come later. For now, sleep.

What are some things that might help you sleep? Reading always makes me fall asleep. I won't take it personally if you don't get to the end of this chapter because reading made you very relaxed . . .

Healthy

Do something good for yourself.

Once you've gone through the eat-whatever-you-want phase, it's time to do something healthy for yourself! It doesn't have to be a sweeping lifestyle change—unless you really want that. Start small. Take a walk, go outside, eat an apple. It also doesn't have to be a physically healthy thing. Paint a picture, go to a museum, see a show, read a book, stimulate your mind.

Inspired

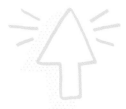

Find inspiration.

Get inspired to make a change—specifically to get out of the gross human slop pile you've created over the past few weeks. I like to watch beauty gurus who are younger than me on YouTube to get inspired to take showers.

Even just thinking about them is making me pissed and somehow motivated. As soon as I'm done writing this chapter, I'm going to do my laundry.

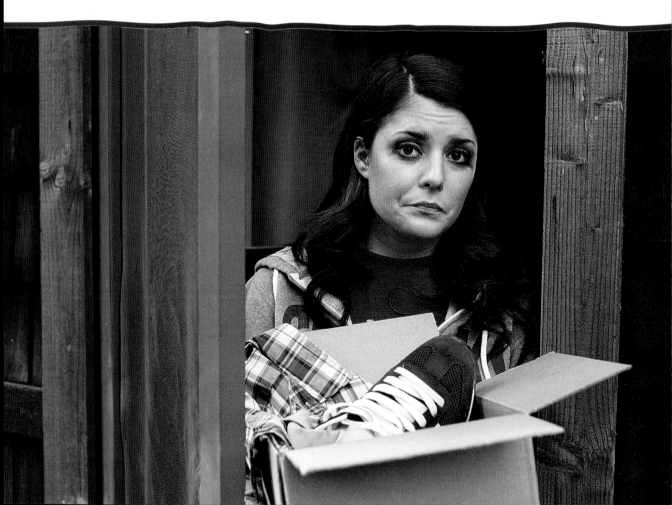

Projects

Use your mind for something other than refreshing your ex's Twitter feed.

What have you been slacking on? What have you wanted to do or been pushing off? Let's get it started. Go team! Now's the time. What else are you going to do? Sit around and wait for your genitals to completely shrivel up? Fun visual! Let's get it going! Go! Go! Go! Also go! And go! And get it! GET IT? I'll stop.

People

Get out of the house and around other humans.

It's probably a good idea to get out of the house and around other people again, but that doesn't mean you have to be particularly outgoing (or even friendly) at first.

There was a period in my life when I first started living in NYC that I got really sad and felt depressed and lonely and I'd force myself to go down to Penn Station to just sit and be around people. I'd observe human behavior and I'd write. What an adorable creep. But it was more helpful than wallowing in my isolation. Also, one of the hallways always smelled like sugar and fresh bagels and I liked that. Eventually, I started improv classes in the city and experienced actual human interaction. That was a nice development.

Go to the grocery store. Go to the park. Baby steps. Just get yourself out there and join

the human race again. It's not all bad.

Entertain

Start entertaining the idea of entertaining.

Or being entertained. Throw a party. Go to a party. Get help from your friends. Have friends invite over other friends you don't know. Go to parties where you don't know everyone. Go out to a concert or comedy show or even a play—whoa.

Let's get you back out there! Get your brain and social skills lubed up. Then maybe you'll get someone else lubed up. LOW FIVE! . . . *moonwalks away* *but then tiptoes back to finish writing this chapter*

Don't

Don't (Internet) stalk your ex.

Don't let yourself fall down the slippery slope of social-media stalking your ex and/or putting yourself in the same physical space as them (as in real-life stalking). You've come a long way—keep your head up and your fingers away from the mouse. You can do this. Move along.

When all is said and done, the only thing that will help you get through a breakup is "time." I know, but it really is true. And don't worry; the sadness truly won't last forever. That sounds like a Celine Dion song. Maybe listen to some Celine Dion. Remember when she wore that backward tuxedo? Hey, you didn't do that. Things are looking up!

Remember:

SAFE SHIPPED

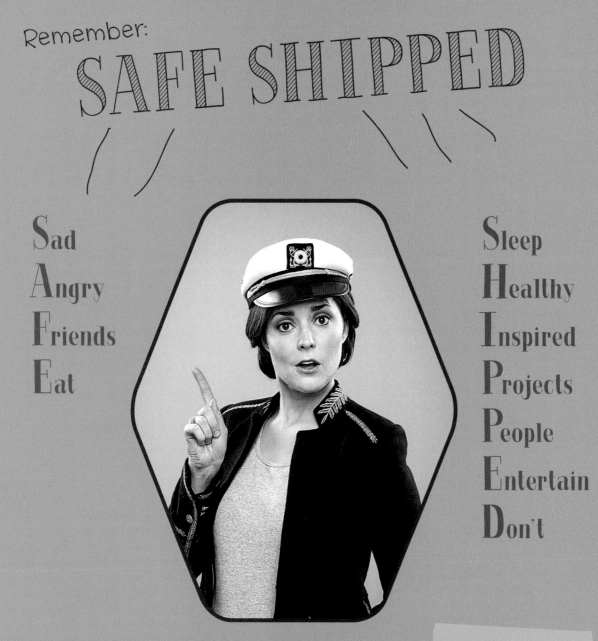

Sad

Angry

Friends

Eat

Sleep

Healthy

Inspired

Projects

People

Entertain

Don't

#SAFESHIPPED

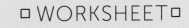

HOW TO SURVIVE
A BREAKUP

Grace notes

DRAW YOUR EX.

DRAW YOUR EX WITH A PENIS
ON HIS/HER FOREHEAD.

DRAW YOUR EX WITH SCROTUMS
FOR ARMS AND LEGS.

DRAW YOUR EX WITH A CHICKEN
STUCK IN HIS/HER BUTT.

DO YOU FEEL ANY BETTER?!?

HOW TO BREAK UP
WITH SOMEONE

There's no "good" way to break up with someone, but there are certainly many horrible ways to do it. Show some respect for the other person. Be honest, give them space afterward, and whatever you do, **don't break up with someone like this**:

1. Publicly. Refrain from breaking up in a place where there are strangers or friends who can hear or see what's happening. Respect the other person enough to let them (potentially) spaz out in private.

2. Over technological devices. Mutual orifices have already been compromised (I assume), so give them the respect of talking out of your mouth hole, in person, to explain your position.

3. Through other people. Don't be a coward. You started this relationship and you're responsible for ending it. You didn't ask your friends to sleep with this person for you, so don't ask them to handle the breakup conversation. I got dumped in seventh grade by a girl who was friends with my boyfriend. She walked into my last-period history classroom before the bell rang to start class, knelt down in front of my desk, and told me that he wanted to break up with me. Before I could reply, she left. And I spent the next forty-five minutes not learning a damn thing about WWII. I hardly knew the girl, but I'll definitely never forget that moment.

THE ART OF ~~JUST COVERING IT IN SPRAY PAINT~~

The Art of Hanging Art, Hanging Out, and Hangovers

THE ART OF CREATING UNIQUE DISHES, ~~INTERESTING SPACES,~~ ~~AND CURES FOR A HANGOVER~~

THE ART OF CURSING OUT HOME
AND FOOD PROGRAMMING

THE ART OF CONVINCING YOURSELF THAT
YOU CAN MAKE THAT THING, TOO

THE ART OF D.I.WHY?

Your Lifestyle

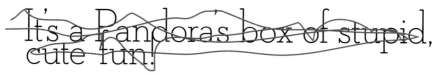
It's a Pandora's box of stupid, cute fun!

This is the lifestyle portion of the book! It's like a sloppy, floppy, hungover HGTV meets a fun-loving, messy Food Network! It's a Pandora's box of stupid, cute fun! Drink every time you read an adjective in this chapter. DON'T. You will die. And I like you. You have neat taste in books.

I've always been enamored with lifestyle stuff. I think a lot of young girls are. It's the combo of reading fashion magazines and watching home improvement shows while simultaneously going through puberty that instills a deep-seated fascination with stylish, pretty things. When I was a teen, I went through the Rolodex of artistic, lifestyle-related careers that I one day hoped to have— magazine editor, travel blogger, journalist, fashion designer, food critic, tiny dog-sleeping-bag maker—until I slowly started to realize that I wasn't fully cut out for those kinds of jobs. There's a certain type-A tidiness and sophistication, both in your organizational skills and your general personal style, that seems to be required for each of those areas. I've always lacked that. No matter how hard I've tried to present myself as a person with her sh*t together, there's an essential sloppiness that's an unshakable part of who I am.

It's taken a long time, but only recently have I embraced this. For instance, I don't remember the last time I've worn jeans. Sweatpants have become my only outfit (MOO). If this is good or bad, I don't know, but I'm, like, so comfortable.

I had my first real eye-opener about my style and sensibility when I decided I wanted to compete in the Miss New Jersey Pageant. I know, I know. I know. Stop. **Most college students are curious about their sexuality, I was curious about what a spray tan felt like.**

Let me explain. Growing up, my step-nana worked in Caesars Casino in Atlantic City, New Jersey, so as kids we grew up going out to dinner and to events for special occasions at the casino. My very first concert was Donnie and Marie Osmond at Caesars. My stepmom took me and a couple of my older cousins and when we were eating dinner she saw Marie walk into the restaurant next to us and had my most agreeable cousin, Matt, run in and get her autograph. It was unsuccessful. One, because the restaurant was crowded, and two, because Matt, being hilariously oblivious, had no idea who Marie was or what she looked like. We also grew up going to the Miss America Pageants and parades that were held in the convention center. I was always in awe of the contestants. I could see my face reflected in their skin. How did they do that?

My older stepcousin, who's now a fitness model in NYC, competed one year and almost won. And since I'm so competitive (see: Tim's foreword), I always thought in the back of my mind that one day I'd compete in a beauty pageant, too. Just to see what it felt like. And win. My parents instilled me with this stupid sense that "You can do anything you put your mind to." Gross.

So sophomore year of college, I applied to the Miss New Jersey competition. Mind you, this pageant was the qualifier to compete for Miss USA, not Miss America. The Miss USA Pageant is kind of like Miss America's less talented stepsister. In fact, there was absolutely no talent portion in the whole competition. It consisted of an opening dance number, introducing yourself over a microphone, and bathing suit and evening-wear rounds. If you made it to the next round, there was a two-minute interview. And that's it.

Anyone could enter, as long as she paid the $1,200 entrance fee. And I did. WHAT WAS I THINKING? I slung so many plates of Applebee's happy hour half-priced boneless buffalo wings for that money. But I had something I needed to prove, I guess.

I didn't tell anyone that I was doing this, except for my boyfriend and my parents. Over the course of the next month, I was on a secret preparation mission. I found a dress at Macy's that was, in hindsight, *very* unflattering. I bought

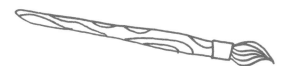

some interview clothes, or what I thought kind of looked like interview clothes, at a Ross Dress for Less. I got spray-tanned and bought fake nails in a shoddy North Jersey salon. I even went online and looked up fake pageant interview questions for practice.

I was there to win. The day before I left for the pageant weekend, my room-mate saw my tacky, shiny blue dress hanging on the back of the door and asked me about it. I finally told her I was doing the Miss New Jersey Pageant and she puked laughter.

"Kaitlyn, I just want *to see!*" I said.

She was a journalism major, so she sort of got it.

The event was at a very posh Hilton Hotel—or as posh as any Hilton I'd seen in Jersey. When I walked through the doors, I felt like I was entering an alternate universe. Perfectly tanned blond girls with their trying-really-hard moms were everywhere. I was by myself holding a dirty Adidas track bag full of clothes. I checked in and was told there was a pizza party that night so everyone could get to know each other. Great.

I was paired in a hotel room with a girl named Candace, who was already watching TV and seemed like she could give two #2's about the whole thing. I liked her. I went to the pizza party and it was . . . something. Clearly, all the girls had just watched *Legally Blonde* and *Miss Congeniality* back-to-back, because everyone was so *outrageously* outgoing. Even with everything I had done to prep, I was not prepared.

I've never seen so many girls under twenty simultaneously try to "work" a room before. I was asked more questions about myself than my boyfriend of a year and a half had ever asked. And, sadly, the pizza was never eaten. I held out for an hour, before I couldn't respond to one more comment of "OMG, you've never been in a pageant before? That's so cute! You're going to have *THE BEST* time." There were some weird psychological *Hunger Games* happening. I went back upstairs and found Candace with three slices of pizza in bed watching reality TV. God, this girl was great.

The next day we learned the opening dance routine—which consisted of a lot of scarf-swirling—and went through a full run of the show. Frantic attempts to win Miss Congeniality continued throughout rehearsals as girls tried to talk to each other about their family hardships and excessively support each other when someone tripped walking offstage. I felt less and less like I had something to prove.

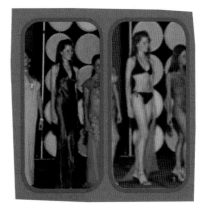

The next morning was the day of the show and everyone was going bonkers. Backstage there was butt tape and spray tans and hairspray like I'd never seen. Yes, I understand why there's a hole in the ozone, environmentalists, I'm very sorry.

I smiled my way through a scarf dance, introduced myself with comical enthusiasm, and wore a bathing suit and evening gown onstage while sporting a "Jersey pouf" hairdo before Snooki was even a thing. Somehow, I made it to the second round and threw on my Ross interview outfit while the other nine girls got sewn into their custom-made skirt suits. I didn't stand a chance. And by that point, I was *SO* okay with that. I answered some questions bluntly, while every other contestant talked about their charity work. OH GOD.

I finished seventh (I think?). But I was first in exiting the building with my parents (who were crazy supportive, even though my dad hates the idea of shallow body-image-based contests). I immediately let them know I never wanted/needed to do that again. I came, I saw, I left right away.

Since this foray into the extreme world of beauty pageants, I've embraced my own awkward, disorderly "grace" (ohhhhhhhh SNAP. BYE) and I've learned how to shape my lifestyle to reflect my personal style and sensibility. Whether it's decorating or cooking or hosting or creating online or recovering from a hangover, here are some strategies to help you live the best life possible. Yay, Oprah!

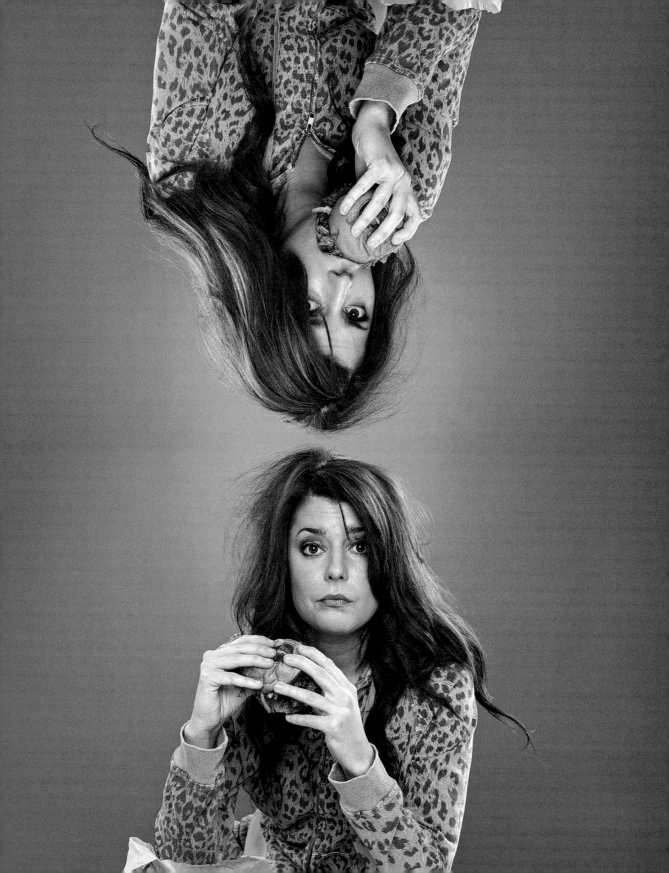

HOW TO
GET
OVER
A
HANGOVER

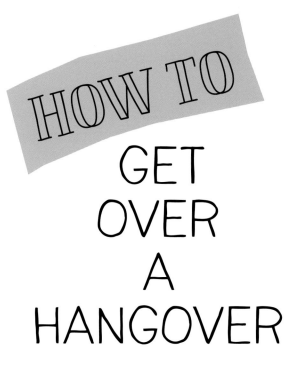

If you currently have a hangover, stop reading this right now. Trying to read when you're hungover is only slightly worse than trying to read when you're sober. #lol #books #irony #stayinschool #unlessschoolisntforyou

Instead, try having a friend read this chapter to you. We'll call your friend "DR." No, not a doctor, a "Designated Reader." But if that person happens to be a doctor, kudos to you for having an intelligent friend who gets paid to touch body parts. Also, maybe ask them how to cure a hangover.

The first step to hangover recovery is accepting that you've brought this upon yourself. If you didn't, you should probably go to the police. Or stop hanging out with Chrissy. I mean, her parents named her Chrissy. Not Christina. Not Christine. Chrissy. A government employee had to print "Chrissy" on a birth certificate. Also, she lets her thong strings show out of the top of her jeggings and she's got a tattoo of a ying-yang on fire. Sorry, but she's bad news.

I've experienced my fair share of hangovers. The first time I got drunk, I was with my best friend at her older sister's college. My high school friend (I'll now refer to her as HSF) had visited a couple of times before and I was desperate to get the college-party experience. I remember thinking, *Jesus, what flared jeans should I wear?*

I was a junior in high school but was a freshman in drinking—and I thought getting drunk was a high school rite of passage. As soon as we got to the dorm, we drank red Solo cups full of pink lemonade and vodka. I was so excited. After just one cup of the sour pink sauce, my face was hot and my body was wiggly. My HSF said, "You'll feel it when you start giggling." I GIGGLED. We walked to my car to grab my overnight bag and it was winter and we laughed like hyenas and kept falling into the dirty gray piles of parking lot snow mountains.

My HSF's sister took us bowling, thinking that a black-light venue with unlimited micro-wave pizza would be a safe space. She was right. Bowling alleys couldn't care less about how you act, as long as you pay for your lane and return their shoes, which smell like dog tongues. HSF's sister also brought a dude friend with her, whose real name we could never remember. Instead my HSF and I decided to call him Lance Bass all night. Why? Because it was an excellent choice. We didn't necessarily call him Lance so much as we just kept repeating the phrase, "Who do you think you are, Lance Bass?" every time he spoke. To us, this was COMEDY GOLD.

It was a great night. We slapped pizza in each other's faces; explained to Lance how we loved *NSYNC in an ironic way, but also like loved them for real; and threw bowling balls overhand down the lanes. I will never forget the image of my HSF drunkenly trying to put pizza in her mouth, but missing and instead smothering her entire face with sauce. I passed out on the floor of my HSF's sister's dorm room and her sister slept next to me all night, because she was worried I wasn't breathing. Turns out I was. Nailed it!

I woke up the next morning and puked into her toilet very politely and drove home with my HSF feeling accomplished and terrible. Over the years, I've put a variety of liquors into my body

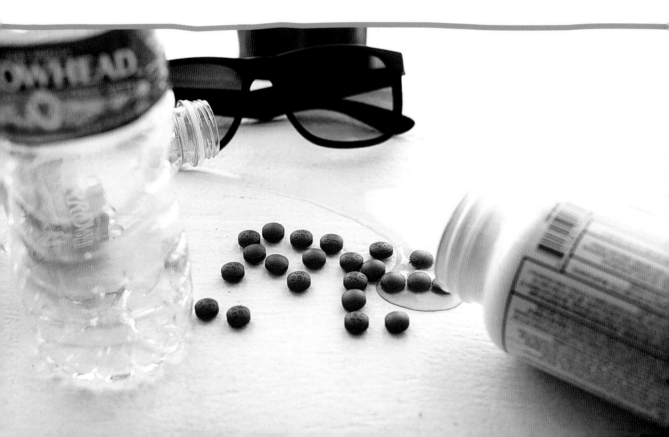

and I've gotten a handle (liquor pun!) on how to manage the inevitable hangover.

It's important to hold yourself accountable even in your sorry state. It will save you unnecessary post-drunk drama and maybe help prevent you from finding yourself in this position again. You're in a sensitive, fleeting state of misery. When you feel terrible, it's incredibly easy to place the blame on someone else. But the truth is, you drank those drinks, you had three "last" shots (I've crowned myself Grace "But shh, let's just do one more shot" Helbig), you hung out with Chrissy. Instead of wasting energy being mad at someone else (or yourself), spend your energy fixing it! Note: You do not have to be happy you did this to yourself; you just have to somehow accept it. PRETEND.

Once you've acknowledged that you are the meteorologist that brought this foggy, bloated haze upon yourself, we can begin.

OKAY, LET'S START THE RECOVERY PROCESS. SORRY I'M SCREAMING.

Drink

Drink the nonpoisons.
Drink water. Take a second and look at the sponge in your kitchen sink right now. Do it. Or if the kitchen is too far away, just Google "dry sponge" or "very old lady." See that? That's your body right now. You are super dehydrated. And YES, duh, I hear you, of course the first thing you should do is drink water—so do it. Get your raggedy, creaky body out of your dirty, makeup-stained sheets and drink it. If not for your health, then for the fact that you can now tell your annoying nonhungover friend, "I already did that, Craig!"

Advil

Take some medicine.
Pop some Advil or some other pain reliever, unless you're one of those holistic, organic, pure people who don't take over-the-counter medicine. In which case, why were you getting so drunk while explaining why Bikram is SO ESSENTIAL? Also, how often do you really clean your yoga mat?

If you're not one of those people, I highly recommend Advil. Again, it seems like common knowledge, I know, but we all need reminders in life. For instance, I keep travel-sized Advil in almost all of my purses/backpacks/suitcases. Some might say that's the sign of a problem, but I say that's the sign of a problem solver.

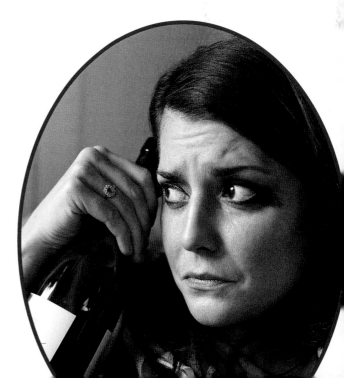

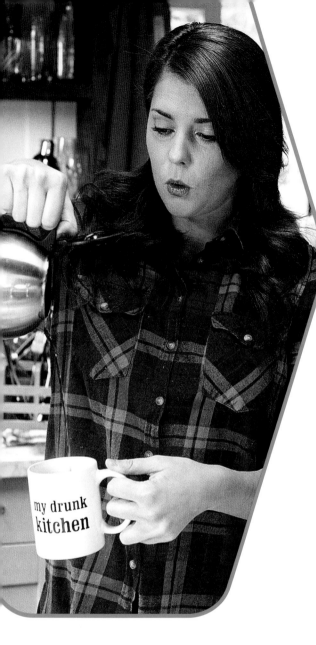

rally, goddamn it. Trust me, it's awful forcing your body out of bed to have lunch at a too-bright Panera Bread with an old college friend, BUT it's extremely wonderful to stay in bed, watch a *Say Yes to the Dress* marathon, and catch up with that old friend's brand-new twins wearing stupid, coordinated striped onesies via Facebook posts. Oh, look at that: the seventeenth photo shows one smiling and the other frowning and they look like human theater masks—SO CUTE. Thanks, Facebook.

heck

Feel up your social media.

Get your hands all over it. This is a big one. Find your phone. Do you have your phone? If you don't, you have a bigger problem. But if you do, tiny congrats. NOW CHECK YOUR INSTAGRAM, TWITTER, FACEBOOK, TUMBLR, VINE, TEXT MESSAGES, OUTGOING CALLS, VOICE MAILS, PHOTO/VIDEO ALBUM. CHECK YOUR LINKEDIN AND MYSPACE PAGES, FOR CHRIST'S SAKE. CHECK IT ALL.

Assess the damage. Figure out what can be salvaged with an "OMG! Kelly stole my phone last night" text or an "I have sinned. I have drunk-tweeted. #blessed" tweet and what cannot be undone. For the actions that may have caused more permanent damage, try not to beat yourself up about it, because it's time to . . .

o

You don't have to do that thing!

Anything you've already planned for the day that can be canceled relatively easily should be canceled. DO IT. You have my permission. Unless it's a Ricky Martin concert—then you

Eat

YEEEEESSSSSS.

This is self-explanatory. All the fries, all the chips,

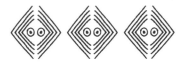

all the huevos rancheros. Go nuts. Give the body what it wants today and don't look back.

Caffeinate

Hit the go-go juice.

If the Advil hasn't cured your headache yet, some coffee might. This step, for me, is key. If you're one of those people who is very sensitive to caffeine, I would hold off—for your sake and the sake of those around you. (I know your type; if you're hungover from a glass and a half of Arbor Mist, the last thing you need is coffee.) But if you're like me, YOU NEED IT.

The good thing about coffee is that it reminds your digestive system that its job is to process both the fries you just ate for brunch and the ones you forgot you ate at three a.m. Oh, yeah . . . those fries.

Revel in Someone Else's Misfortune (Schadenfreude)

Things could be so much worse.

Your present state is way okay because it could be SO MUCH WORSE. Sometimes, it's helpful to look up the Kony2012 guy's public breakdown and let yourself relive those few moments of raw joy and raw pain and raw nudity. Other times, it's nice to take a few minutes/hours to look at your ex-boyfriend's photos on Instagram and confirm that his beard DEFINITELY looks stupid. And his facial hair is pretty bad, too. HEYO.

Personally, I love watching marathons of *Chopped* and *Toddlers and Tiaras* when I'm

QUICK REMINDERS

- This will **NOT** last forever.
- You're not dying. Unless you have some disease you didn't tell me about. In which case, I defer to your doctor friend.
- As long as you did not tell someone you love to "eat poop" or someone you do **NOT** love to "eat me," everything is going to be okay. Celebrate! Pop the champ . . . water bottle!

hungover. I like to indulge myself by watching shows with very few winners.

One

One is the best number.

Try to do just one good thing for yourself today. When your body is feeling miserable, it's easy for your brain to follow the depression train to bummer station. Instead! Trick your brain into thinking you're still okay by doing something relatively healthy and maybe productive. Start a project you've been putting off, do a goddamn DIY project you saw on Pinterest, masturbate, etc.

When I wake up hungover, or come home from a long weekend of drinking, I like to order juice cleanses online. It makes me feel like I'm Jennifer Aniston. And she's doing okay—now. Usually by the time I get the delivery of juices I'm

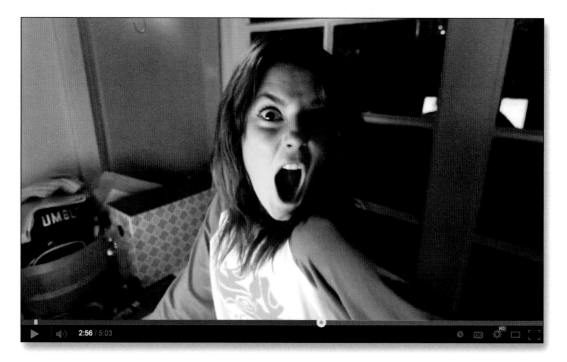

like, "Da fuq?" But in that very hungover moment of ordering them, I feel better.

Tumblr

Don't retch, reblog.

Tumblr is a wonderful distraction from the post-drinking, self-hating nausea-panic caused by hangovers.

Clean

Yes, yes, I want some scrubs . . .

Clean yourself. Take a long, hot shower. Imagine the guilt, anxiety, and dance-sweat rinsing off you. It's fun to try to scrub away the bad memories. Showers can be magical. Play some music, sing into the showerhead, pee—let it all out.

Hair

Dogs are great. And hair of the dog is the best.

If you haven't already done so, it's time to give your body a little bit of the midnight poison. I don't think midnight poison is an actual term for alcohol, but it is now! Fun! It's like that age-old saying, what doesn't kill you . . . makes its way into a Bloody Mary and reduces your hangover panic attack.

This is a personal preference, but I find it's better to ease my body down from a mountain of booze with a little more booze. It's like when people run a marathon and then do some cool-down jogging afterward and you think, *We get it, you LOVE running, stop showing off.* Hair of the dog is your post-marathon jog. You're very athletic.

Remember:

DANCE CROTCH

Drink

Advil

No

Check

Eat

Caffeinate

Revel in Someone Else's Misfortune (Schadenfreude)

One

Tumblr

Clean

Hair

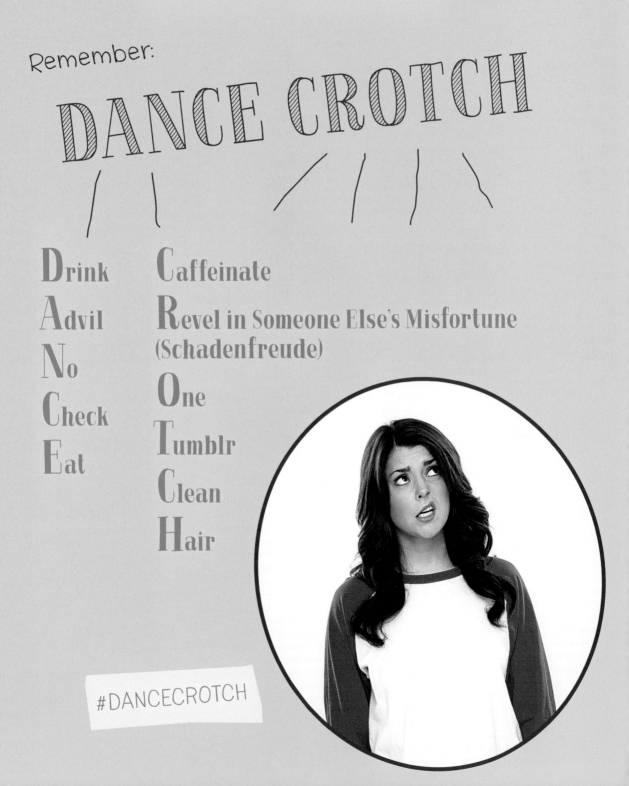

#DANCECROTCH

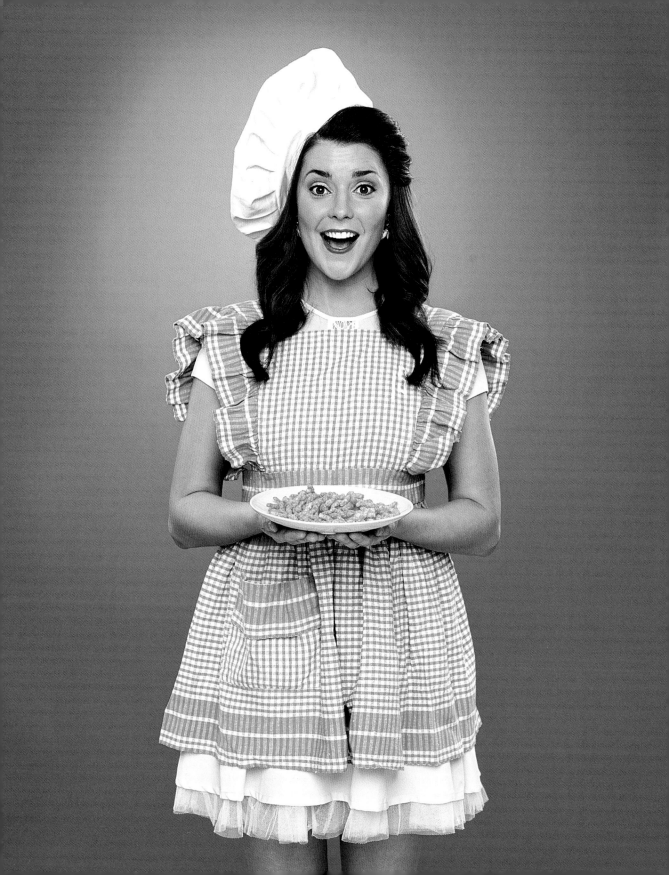

HOW TO
COOK
LIKE
A KID
FOR
ADULTS

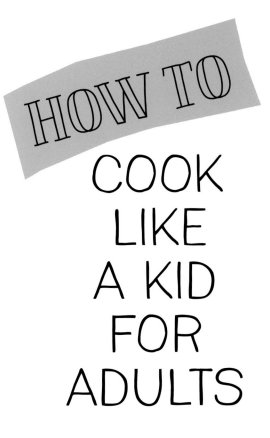

I'm not a good cook. Clearly. This is something I've come to understand and accept about myself. I have limitations. I've tried at various points in my life to leverage my obsession with the Food Network to raise my cooking game and it never works. I have the cooking abilities of a college freshman. I understand how to work with a small group of basic foods and products, and anything beyond that is too much. Foodies intimidate and terrify me. But when I imagine what a life based around a truffle-oil obsession must be like, I laugh. So dumb.

When I moved to NYC, I was scared of "fancy" restaurants. I didn't know anything about wine (other than that a $12 bottle from the liquor store down the street was a splurge for me). If the menu items were in another language, I was royally screwed (I was too intimidated to ask questions, and if I did, I didn't understand the answers). And all I really ever wanted at the end of the day was cheap, sloppy Mexican food and a margarita. There's gotta be at least one other person out there who feels the same way—so this chapter is for you!

Just because my cooking knowledge is elementary doesn't mean I can't try to invent creative dishes. Foodies can't hold me down (mostly because I don't think they have the upper body strength). Yes, these recipes might not be the greatest for your body, but they're fun to make. And that's half of what I think is so appealing about cooking—the process.

Tools and utensils your starter-kitchen needs

- A handwritten list of your close friends and family members' phone numbers stored in a drawer for when you spill a pot of boiling water on your phone.
- Some sort of cleaning products to wipe off the gross.
- Objects that can be used to put out potential fires.
- Chips.
- Something for stirring things (professional note: don't use fountain pens).
- Knives (mostly regular-sized, but maybe one intimidatingly big one in case someone breaks into your house and you need to protect yourself and be like, "DON'T STEAL MY STUFF I HAVE A GIANT KNIFE!").
- PAM or other nonstick sprays—the dry shampoo of cooking.
- Some sort of heating tool and heating chambers (oven, microwave, grill, skillets, etc.). (Side joke: Who is a skillet, a grill, and my ex-boyfriend's favorite musician? . . . Skrillex—BYE.)
- Probably some bowls.

BREAKFAST

Huevos Ranch-OOOHs

This is a GREAT hangover meal and it combines the culinary traditions of Mexico and Pittsburgh. Mexico is known for the classic dish huevos rancheros and Pittsburgh is known for putting french fries on sandwiches. This is the meal for the person who wants some sloppy Mexican in the morning, but also can't stop thinking about that side of fries. Why not force them to mingle? That's how real friends are made! Also, there's ranch dressing on this because fries and ranch dressing go together like Spanx and a tight dress.

Ingredients:

- Frozen french fries
- Taco seasoning
- Beans (black or refried—you'll be the one farting them out later, so pick whichever is most pleasing to you)
- Tortillas
- Eggs
- Ranch dressing
- Salsa
- Cilantro (if you're fancy)
- Salt and pepper

Cook your french fries according to the package's instructions (but sprinkle them with some taco seasoning before you put them in the oven). Heat your beans and tortillas while you cook your eggs any way you want. You could go the apathetic route and use a microwave or be quasi-impressive and heat the beans in a skillet and warm your tortillas over your stovetop burners to get a little char (I told you I watch the Food Network). Cook your eggs however you want. When everything has been heated, start reverse-Jenga stacking! Lay down your tortillas, throw on some beans, add some fries, smother with some ranch dressing, top with your eggs and salsa. If you're fancy, chop up some cilantro and put it on top. Done! You now have a delicious Mex-sylvania breakfast! You did it!

Changing of the Carbs

Like the changing of the guards? In England? Whatever. This recipe gives an ENGLISH muffin a whole new meaning. Hot damn! This is for someone who likes fish sandwiches and also likes salt-and-vinegar chips. Are there people like that out there? This is a conceptual dish if you're the kind of person that prefers quirky titles over actual taste. Because, honestly, I've never made this, but it sounds decent in theory. And when it comes to food, decent is okay by me!

One of the most well-known English dishes is fish-and-chips (which is usually fried fish and French fries). It's great. It hits all the spots. Sometimes it comes with tartar sauce, sometimes malt vinegar, sometimes curry sauce. This recipe is a spin on that classic.

Ingredients:

- ☐ Fish sticks (or fish or frozen fish)
- ☐ English muffin
- ☐ Tartar sauce (or make your own if you're one of those people)
- ☐ Salt-and-vinegar chips
- ☐ Lettuce (optional)

Cook up the fish sticks according to the package's instructions. (Or attempt to batter and fry your own fish if you have something to prove. Honestly, battering and frying your own fish will probably taste better, so I salute you.) Toast your English muffin. Now it's time to build the sandwich. Slather (what a word) the muffin with tartar sauce, smash in some salt-and-vinegar chips, pile on the fish and lettuce (if you want) and you're done! Taste it to see if it doesn't completely suck. Cool job!

Spamcakes

This is a pretty straightforward dish. It's pancakes with Spam in them. If you don't know what Spam is, you're really missing out. If bacon and sausage had a super-white-trash daughter, it'd be Spam. It's salty and savory and what exact meat it actually is remains unknown. It's like a game for your mouth! Except don't think about the last part for too long or you'll gross yourself out. Some might call it "Hot Dog's Cousin" or "Scrapple's Stepdad." Because sometimes in the morning you want something salty and sweet.

There was a period in my life after college when I was eating pancakes for dinner EVERY NIGHT. After a long shift at the good ol' Olive Garden slopping six-pound plates of pasta swimming in Alfredo sauce, coming home to one giant pancake was perfect. They were cheap, they were filling, and they were transformable. They were like edible paper dolls that you could dress up with different fillings and toppings. Cute!

Ingredients:

- ☐ Spam
- ☐ Vegetable oil or PAM
- ☐ Pancake mix (or you can make your pancakes from scratch if you want to, oof)
- ☐ Water or milk (depending on the mix you bought)
- ☐ Butter or syrup (your choice)

Chop or dice your Spam into smaller pieces and sauté them in a pan with oil or PAM until they're to your liking (hint: unlike hair, crispy Spam is great Spam). Mix your pancake mix together and then add your cooked Spam. Set another skillet up with a buttered bottom (ha) and ladle your mixture into the pan to cook your pancakes. Make them as big or little as you'd like but make sure they're cooked through. How do you know if they're cooked through? The same way you annoy someone on Facebook—poke them. See if stuff oozes out.

LUNCH

Hot Dog Salad

For those of you out there watching your figure but don't give an expletive about being refined, this dish is for you! It's like wearing an evening dress with Uggs; it's the tuxedo T-shirt of food.

First of all, hot dogs are delicious. I just recently started eating meat again after seven years as a pescetarian, and five days into my new meat-eating lifestyle, I had bone marrow. Meh. Then I had a hot dog. SWEET LORD. How could I have deprived myself of this simple joy? But at the same time, when I was a pescatarian, my favorite fake meat was the veggie dogs. So this dish can work both ways! Equal opportunity food!

At the end of the day, I'm still a lady and I want to try to convince myself that I'm putting decent edibles into my body. Cue: salad!

Ingredients:

□ Hot dogs (regular or veggie)
□ Hot dog rolls
□ Salad fixings (whatever you like, I don't know you)

□ Olive oil
□ Honey mustard dressing
□ Pickles and/or relish

This is basically like a deconstructed hot dog. "Deconstructed" is a neat, pretentious word that all those fancy food people like to use. First, you're going to cook your hot dogs however you prefer. Grill, George Foreman, boil, oven, whatever. The world is your oyster dog. While that cooks, chop up the hot dog buns into cubes as best you can and cook them in a skillet with some olive oil—we're making croutons out of them! EXPLETIVE! While both are cooking, prep your salad any way you prefer. When the hot dogs are done, chop them up and add them to the salad with your croutons and toss the whole thing with honey mustard (BECAUSE MUSTARD GOES ON HOT DOGS) and relish (optional—just thought it kept in line with the theme, but MAYBE I'M WRONG, Jesus Christ). Enjoy!

Macachos

This recipe is a classic. It's one of the first cooking videos I ever put up on the Internet. It's the simplest of stupid meals. And perfect for those who have not yet developed digestive issues. Fundamentally, it's nachos with mac and cheese as the cheese. When I conceptualized this I thought to myself, *How can I make a terrible meal more terrible? Add more carbs and dairy!* Done! Yay, creativity! Boo, arteries!

Ingredients:

□ Mac and cheese
□ Tortilla chips

Whatever you like on your nachos—including but not limited to:

□ Beans

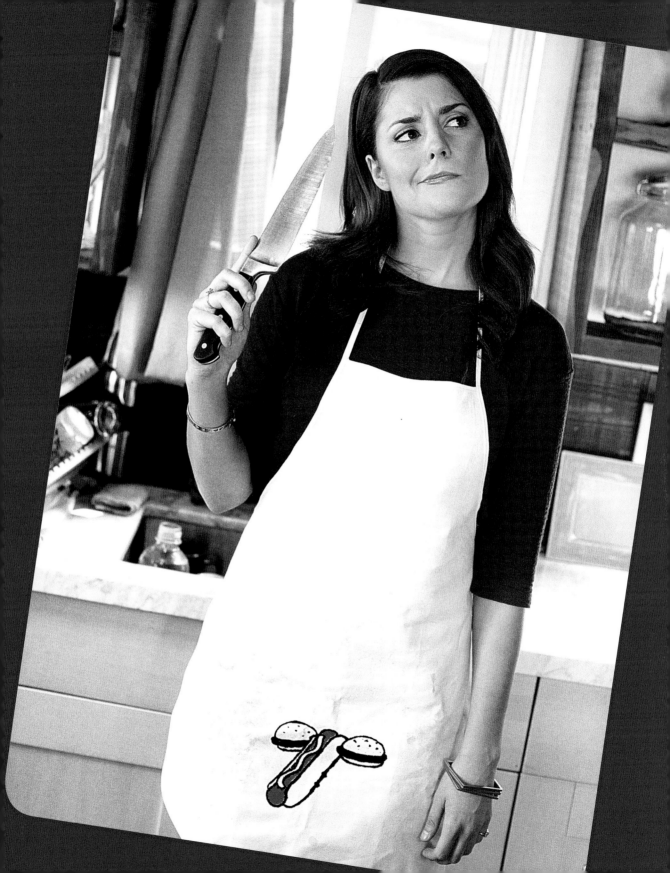

- ☐ Tomatoes
- ☐ Jalapeños
- ☐ Onions
- ☐ Corn
- ☐ Cilantro
- ☐ Salsa
- ☐ Sour cream
- ☐ Avocados/guacamole

Cook your mac and cheese according to the box's directions. Unless you want to make some from scratch so the rest of us look like incompetent fart factories. Thanks. Let the mac and cheese cool while you toast your tortilla chips. This is the sneak-attack part of nachos—tortilla chips with burnt edges. Sweet deity in a Babybjörn, they're good. Feel free at this point to heat up your beans if you're a hot beans person. Hot Beans is a great name for a child. Once the mac and cheese and tortillas have had a chance to cool, start assembling. This is up to you, but I usually layer the chips, mac and cheese, beans, and the rest of the stuff that's going to blow out of my butthole. Butt appetit!

Charade-uterie

I've only recently learned this, but "charcuterie" is basically a plate of fancy meat that a lot of swanky restaurants serve. According to Wikipedia it's prepared meat products, such as bacon, ham, sausage, terrines, galantines, pâtés, and confit, primarily from pork. Yes, those are actual words that mean something and not just hands slamming on the keyboard to produce a series of letters. Very sophisticated. But it's easy to create the poor man's pseudo-charcuterie, or the charade-uterie.

Ingredients:
- ☐ Meat (any meat you want from your grocery store's deli section; it doesn't have to be cured; bologna, pepperoni, honey-glazed ham, smoked turkey, etc., will do)
- ☐ Mustard or dipping sauces
- ☐ Olives or pickles
- ☐ A tray

Take all of the ingredients and slap them onto a tray in a way that doesn't look like it fell on the floor and then you tried to pick everything back up in a hurry. Perfect.

DINNER

Palzone

This dish will always be there for you. It has a lot of the things you want in a pal: it's simple, but has layers, it has great taste, and is always a little saucy. It's a calzone full of pasta. Cue the Spice Girls: when two become oooooone. It promises to be a crowd favorite, especially for a crowd about to participate in an Iron Man competition, because it's a WHOLE LOTTA carbs.

Ingredients:
- ☐ Pasta (whichever you prefer)
- ☐ Sauce (again, whatever you prefer)
- ☐ Cheese (SERIOUSLY, whatever you prefer)
- ☐ Protein (optional/OMG IT'S WHATEVER YOU PREFER)
- ☐ Pizza dough (prepackaged or look up how to make your own—how helpful of me)
- ☐ Flour
- ☐ Olive oil

Preheat your oven to about 450 degrees. Boil your water, add your pasta, cook through, drain, and let cool. If you're using protein, cook it to your liking while you heat your sauce. After they're all done, mix the pasta, sauce, and protein together. Spread out your dough on a flat, floured surface and add the pasta mixture to one half of the dough (leaving about an inch of crust on the outside). Add your cheese on top of the pasta. Fold the crust over the mixture like a doughy sleeping bag and crimp the ends together with a fork. Add a little olive oil on top and place it on a floured baking sheet or pizza stone (that thing you've had for five years but haven't used yet!). Let it cook for ten to fifteen minutes or until the dough is golden brown—like a sixty-year-old divorcee in Key West. Bring it out of the oven, let it cool, and see if it tastes like food! God bless!

Mashed Potstickers

This is maybe the easiest and most stoner-appropriate recipe so far. I didn't intend on it being this way, but it's going to be delicious. I think. This is something I actually haven't made before, but in my head it sounds pretty neat. This isn't necessarily a full dinner, more of a side. But it's probably not the best for you (even though there are some vegetables in there!) and you might end up eating more than you originally thought, so let's assume it's a dinner and call it a relatively guilt-free night (even though we both know you're going to wake up in the middle of the night and eat the cold leftovers—treat yo'self!).

Ingredients:

☐ Frozen potstickers (or make your own, hippie)
☐ Instant mashed potatoes (or make your own, yuppie)

☐ Soy sauce (optional)
☐ Sriracha (optional)

Heat the potstickers according to the directions on the packet. Or however your homemade-loving butt makes them. Allow them to cool while you make your instant potatoes (or first start by boiling your potatoes to make mashed potatoes from scratch before you make your potstickers, if you're one of those). Once your potatoes are finished and cooling, mash up your potstickers as much as you can and blend them into the potato mix. Add soy sauce and Sriracha to taste! You did it! You're a cultural icon!

DESSERT

Ice-Cream Bamwich

This is a savory sweet treat that's sure to satisfy the mature child in all of us. It's pretty simple, and guaranteed to please even your most uptight foodie friend, Eben (with a *b*), who thinks any type of "sandwich" for dessert is juvenile. F you, Eben.

Ingredients:

☐ Cookies
☐ Bacon
☐ Vanilla ice cream (or whatever you want—have you not gotten this by now?)

Feel free to make cookies or buy cookies. Whatever you prefer. Cook the bacon to a crispy, fatty finish. God, bacon is the best. While the bacon rests, warm your cookies in the oven (if they're premade). Then construct your sandwich. In between two warm cookies stack vanilla ice cream and bacon, and BOOM, GODDAMN, SEE YOU TOMORROW, EBEN!

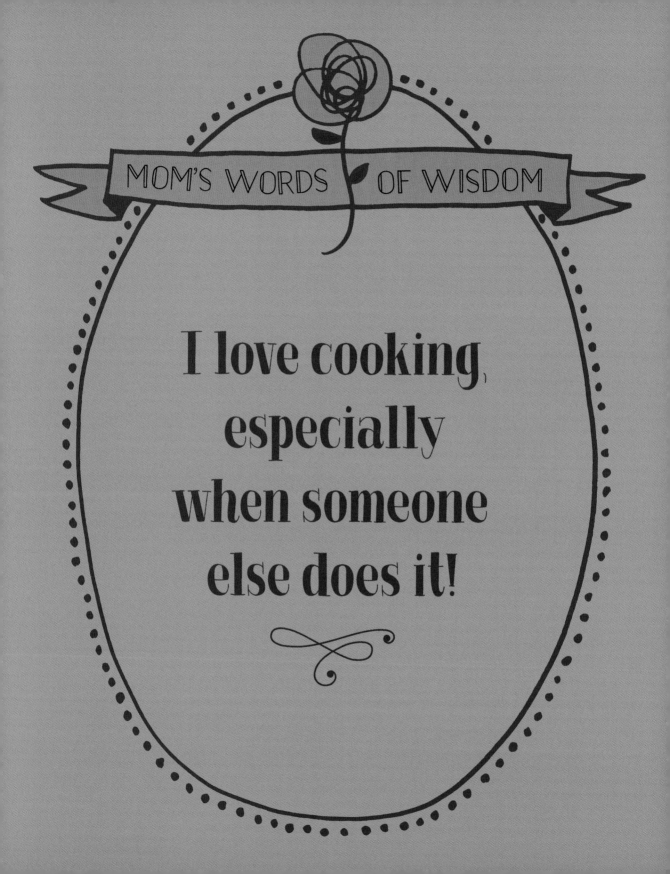

MOM'S WORDS OF WISDOM

I love cooking, especially when someone else does it!

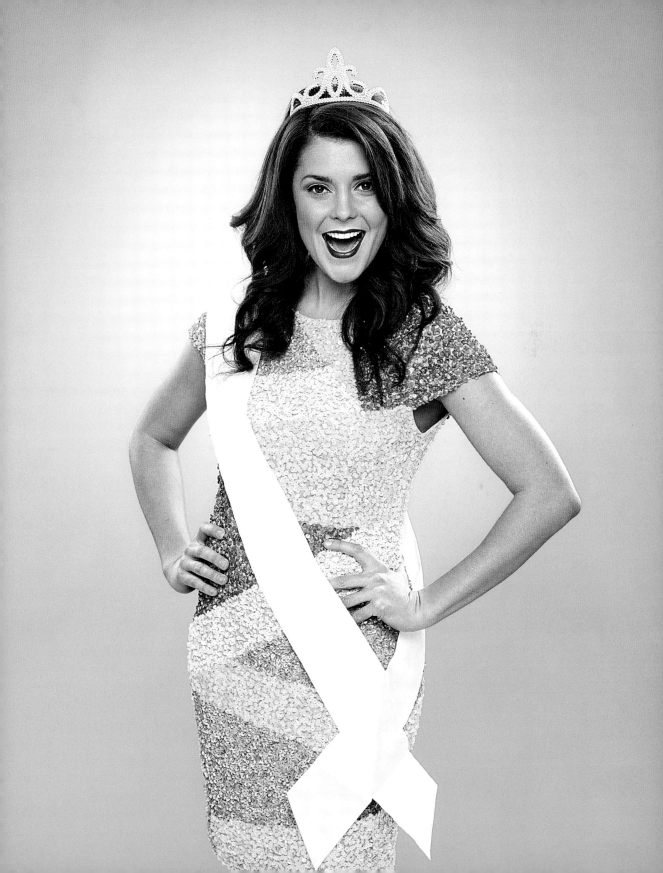

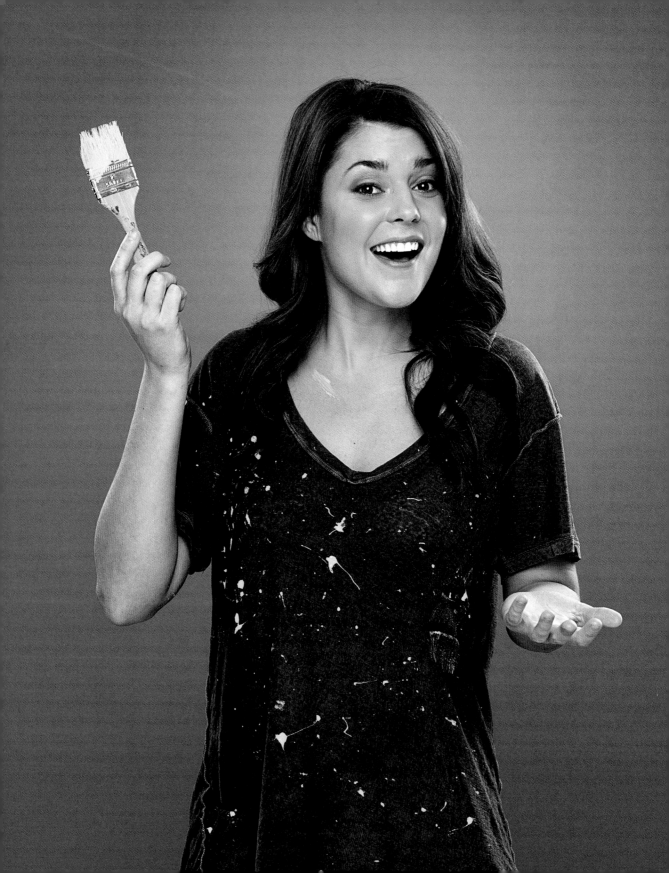

HOW TO
DECORATE LIKE AN ADULT

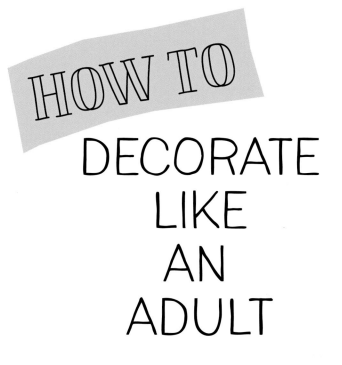

I've been obsessed with interior design since I was in middle school. I would binge-watch TLC's *Trading Spaces* and anything on HGTV until my eyes couldn't take another crown molding face-lift. When I was growing up, my mom would let me redo my bedroom once every five years or so and I would go nuts. Cue the makeover montage!

I would sift through pages and pages AND PAGES of a JCPenney's catalog to find the PERFECT wall unit with a twin bed frame attached. I would experiment with floral and cheetah-print bedding to complement my extensive (but sophisticated) stuffed animal and porcelain doll collection.

When I was a senior in high school I thought it would be super "rad" to paint my walls neon green. It was also the year my parents gave me my first used desktop computer, so I LIVED on the Internet in my room. I spent an entire year living in a green screen, convincing myself it was chic and edgy and wasn't the reason I couldn't sleep at night.

The most exciting part about going to college wasn't picking my major or making new friends; it was choosing my DORM DESIGN SCHEME! And trust me, if you're shopping for your dorm room gear, Target will ruin you. They know exactly what they're doing. My dorm rooms were usually around two feet by two feet. Did I really need that tiny bean-bag chair that matched my mouse pad? No! But YES. They got to me.

My style was restricted in college, because I knew I'd be moving into a new space with new rooms and new area-rug possibilities the next semester. That philosophy traveled with me after I graduated and moved into a series of crappy apartments in Brooklyn with my college roommate. Those terrible apartments let our terrible design skills shine.

In our first apartment, my roommate's bedroom theme was pink. She had two pink curtains, a pink duvet, and in the daytime when the light shined in, it turned her whole room pink. My boyfriend at the time thought her theme was Inside of a Vagina. Meanwhile, I was rocking a twin-lofted bed with a small desk underneath. You can take the girl out of college but you can't take the space-saving furniture out of the girl, because Brooklyn apartments are tiny and expensive.

When we moved to our next apartment with overly embellished, brownish laminate-tiled floors, we thought we could paint the walls dynamic colors to distract from the faded flooring and popcorn ceiling. The more stuff we hung, the worse it looked. It was a disaster from the start. But it was fun!

I ended up moving many more times in the next year and adopted an if-I-got-it-at-IKEA-it's-part-of-a-purposeful-design philosophy. The place I finally ended up staying in for about three years was a true post-college, freshman-year-of-life apartment. It was a great space, but there was no design scheme. I bought a few bold pieces from IKEA and mixed them with some free stuff people left in the lobby of my building and tried to complement that with what I thought were "quirky" self-drawn art pieces to create a bohemian chic feel. It was more like bohemian-ick. In the back of my mind I still thought that I'd move out of this place at any point and I shouldn't invest in furniture or real decoration. Yeeeah, that's what I thought. Suuuure.

When I moved to Los Angeles I ended up finding a place that had so much potential for coolness that it would have been an affront to

the design gods if I didn't at least try to make it look kewl and neat and hip. So I got rid of almost everything I had in Brooklyn and started fresh. I filled the place with flea market finds and throw pillows and a taxidermied hamster butt.

After visiting a lot of friends' and strangers' places out in LA (and on Pinterest), I've gotten a handle on decorating like an adult—simply and cheaply. So here are some of the tips I've picked up over the past few years. Take them or defecate on them, I don't care.

Flea Markets

So much better than real fleas.

When I was younger my mom used to take us to flea markets so we could get specialized T-shirts that said something like YOU KNOW YOU'RE ITALIAN WHEN . . . or YOU KNOW YOU'RE A GYMNAST WHEN . . . (I really wanted everyone to know I was a gymnast) and the shirts would list a bunch of HILARIOUS stereotypes like, YOU KNOW YOU'RE ITALIAN WHEN YOUR COLOGNE IS MARINARA SAUCE. Solid gold. God, I'd love to meet the person who designed those shirts. But that was my only flea market association until I became an adult.

As an adult I think flea markets are THE SHIZZ (you say that, right?). It's like when you're a preteen and you realize you can get Calvin Klein jeans at Ross Dress for Less in your price range and you're all like, *Look at me, fellow tweens, I'm sophisticated as hell*. That's what flea markets are for adults.

I've been able to find so many cool things for a cheap price that make it look like I've been visited by a CB2 fairy in the night. The best part about flea markets is that (usually) you

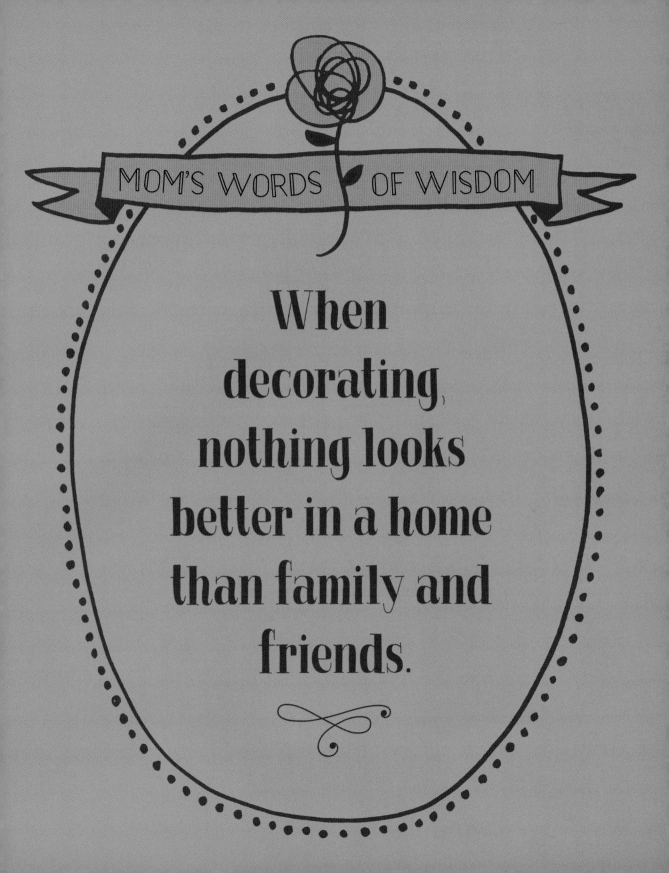

MOM'S WORDS OF WISDOM

When decorating, nothing looks better in a home than family and friends.

What your candle scent says about you

Fresh laundry: You hardly ever do your laundry.

Lavender: One time like a bunch of years ago you read something in a book you can't remember or someone that you can't remember told you that lavender, like, really relaxes you. It's a fact.

Vegetable scents: You really, really want to be interesting (but seriously, a tomato vine candle smells GREAT—I hate myself).

Most fruit scents: You have three children and love appletinis.

Coconut: You've had a threesome.

Vanilla/other sugary scents: You've never tried it up the butt but if you got drunk enough you'd probably do it.

Grass/wood scents: You're a man but are curious about candles.

Peach: You're constipated.

Any drink scent: A half glass of Arbor Mist gets you blackout.

Ocean/weather/seasonal scents: You were cool in high school and now you kind of suck.

can negotiate the prices. So even for the softest of hearts it's a fun environment to pretend for a moment that you're a hardass. "Fifty dollars? I'll give you forty-eight." Done deal, you ruthless, money-sucking vampire who covets mid-century furniture. Good for you.

IKEA

More like Ike-duh!

Sometimes you just can't beat it. They have everything. And they have it in a price range you can probably afford. Yes, it'll take years off your life putting it together, but afterward you'll feel a sense of accomplishment right before you realize you somehow have three leftover screws that shouldn't be left over. But at least now you have that lime-green dresser you've always sort of wanted!

I used to try to decorate my apartment with almost all IKEA furnishings—and you could tell. Now I find it's fun to mix and match IKEA products and flea market finds with a couple of more expensive splurge items. Also, that sentence is the intro to my new HGTV show *Re-decor-GRACE*. It's a working title.

Scents

Candles, candles, candles!

I've become obsessed with candles. I can't help it. The Bath and Body Works two-for-$20 deal always gets me. And they have so many scents! Yes, inevitably they all smell like sugar, but some of them are different. I've even done the thing where I look for coupon codes online just to get more of a discount. TLC has really started to affect me (the television station, not the girl band).

I feel that candles and pleasant scents give the illusion of a clean home, even if your area is a scum palace. Same for food: if it smells good, you'll probably eat it. Maybe that's just me. Maybe that's why my stomach is a horror show with no intermission. Anyway, candles are an easy, relatively cheap way to trick people into thinking your place is chicer than it is. Also, I think I heard one time that candles are cool for relaxing, specifically if you're a person who enjoys taking baths and soaking in your own human soup. Cool for you.

Portland and collectively they cost ten dollars. What a steal! USA! USA! USA! Also since they're from Portland, they're especially weird and kewl. Humble brag. But putting them on the wall by themselves looked kind of tacky, so I went to—you guessed it—IKEA and found three simple wood frames for ten dollars each. Now the posters look expensive and stylish. Or at least I think so. At the end of the day, you can only please yourself. But seriously, try frames.

Hang It

Give your walls friends!

Posters were a key part of my style when I was younger. I put posters on my bedroom walls, in my locker, in my dorm room, and all of my friends had posters, too. It was a cheap, easy way to express myself. As an adult, I've graduated to using actual picture frames. Whoa. Who knew? Some people knew.

I can still express myself by hanging what I consider to be "art," but now it looks more expensive and purposeful. I recently bought three posters when I was up in

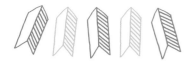

You Could Make That

DIY is very "now."

There's a lot of stuff sold at ridiculous prices in stores that can be made on the cheap. Curtains and decorative pillows are definitely easy DIY projects. I made a decorative pillow out of a Boy Scout uniform one time. It's cute and creepy.

Even though sites like Pinterest and Etsy are sometimes over the top, they're great for inspiring your own creativity. Sometimes I impress myself with my DIY skills and sometimes I look back on a project and think, *Da fuq?* Like the time I drew a cartoon Mona Lisa thinking of a hamburger and put it in a frame made of pool-noodle foam I found in the children's section of IKEA. Some DIY ideas become DI-WHY?

Green Things

Plants!

Plants make a house feel like a house with plants in it! They're great! I've only recently learned their value after moving to California, where "lush" isn't just a store that sells soap—everything grows here. I used to think plants were like children, cool in theory but just a pain in the ass to keep alive, until I found succulents and cacti! They're almost impossible to kill! It's opened up a whole new world of possibility for me. They look cool and come in a ton of different shapes and sizes and colors. And you can use your DIY imagination to plant them in all sorts of unusual objects and place them in clusters and groups. They're a boring person's fail-safe decorating tool.

If you're better than the rest of us and can actually keep some plants alive, go for the hard stuff. Adding green to your space is calming and makes people think you're stylish and functional. Decorating, as most of the rest of life, is all about appearances. And the Benjamins, or so I've heard.

Rugs

Give your floor a hat!

Just like frames, rugs are a great tool to spice up your space. Think of them as floor frames or floor hats. Even an inexpensive rug can help express your personal style and tie the other elements in the room together. Oh, what's that? YOU JUST GOT RE-DECOR-GRACED! It doesn't roll off the tongue as well as I'd hoped.

There's not much else to say about rugs other than that I support them, they're easy to swap out to refresh a room's design scheme, and just like me, they let people walk all over them. How much better could they be?

Over Time

Like an elderly person crossing the street, good design happens slowly.

I've always been one to move into a new space and immediately want to buy EVERYTHING I need to fully decorate it in one day—or as soon as humanly possible. And that's not always the best philosophy. You can find really great pieces if you give yourself time to look. Don't settle for something just because you want to fill your space fast. That is, unless someone is holding you at gunpoint and really, really needs you to

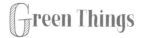

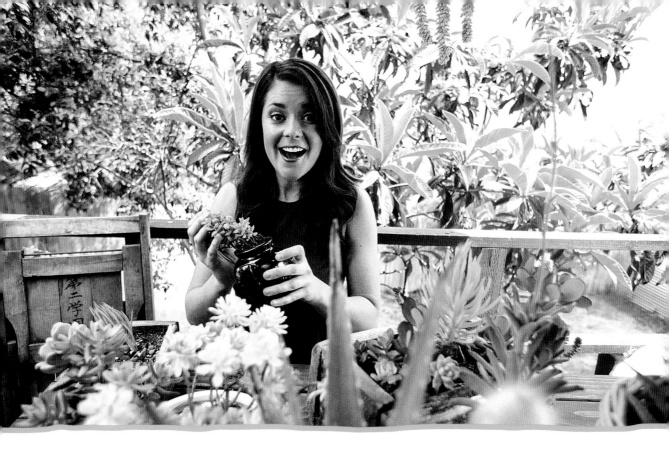

pick an area rug, then go with the blue one with the squiggles. Otherwise, don't rush.

It took me weeks to find the right taxidermied hamster butt on Etsy, but eventually I did. And it lives proudly above my back door. The butt door.

Paint

"Paint" rhymes with "taint"!

You can take a crappy piece of furniture and turn it into a happy piece of furniture with paint! Spray paint, chalk paint, paint paint—there are a lot of ways you can transform old items with paint. Before you pass up on a piece of furniture with great bones or get rid of a much-loved object already in your home, see if there's a way to refurbish it. Imagine your dresser is the face of a desperate fifty-year-old Beverly Hills socialite,

layer on the makeup, and give those drawers some cougar appeal!

Experiment

Get wild, you weirdo!

It's just like how you experimented in college with Krysten (with a *y*) and that foreign exchange student, except completely different. There will be no pickles in this version. You were weird in college.

Experiment with your design. Find your aesthetic and let your creativity run wild. See what happens. If you don't like it, you can change it! That's the beauty of decorating. Unlike tattoos and plastic surgery, it's a creative way to express yourself that isn't permanent! Can't say the same about your Garfield tramp stamp. Eesh.

Remember:
FISHY GROPE

Flea Markets   **G**reen Things

IKEA   **R**ugs

Scents   **O**ver Time

Hang It   **P**aint

You Could Make That   **E**xperiment

#FISHYGROPE

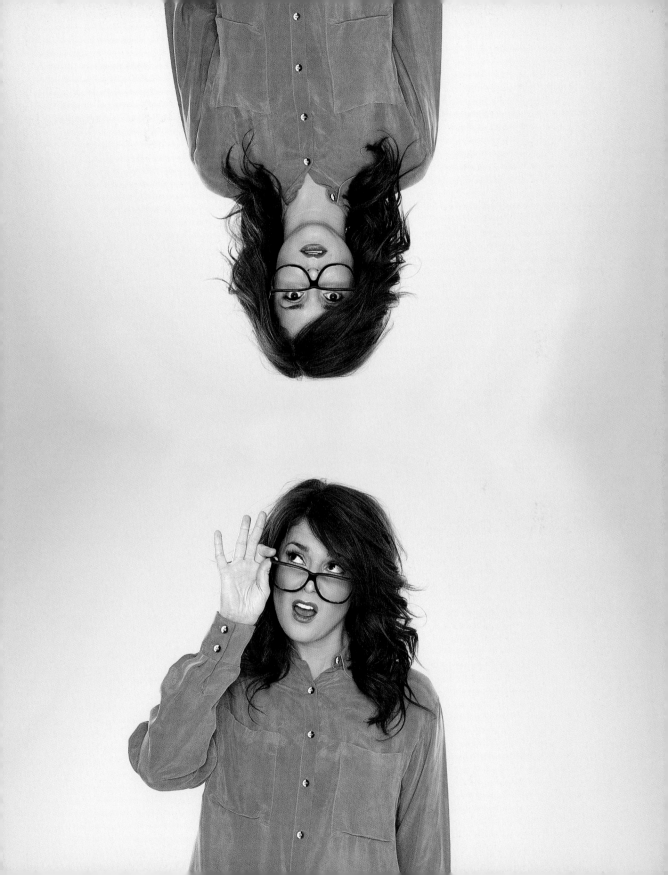

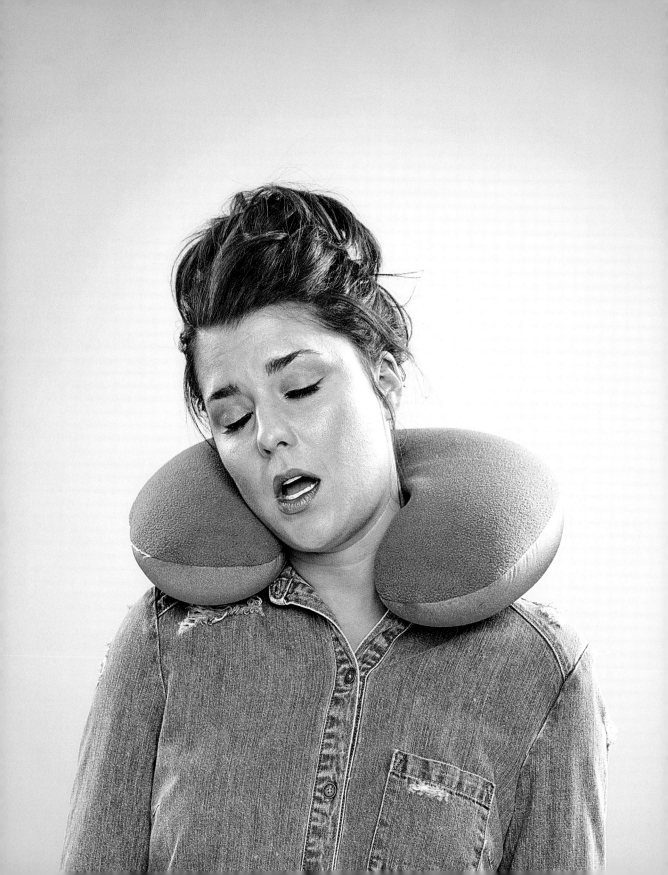

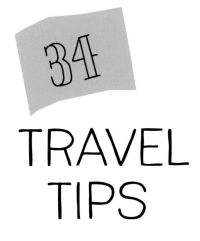

TRAVEL TIPS

Traveling is the best. Unless you're agoraphobic, then it's the worst. I get that. I can't fix that for you. I'm sorry. But for the people who like to travel, let's talk.

I've increased the amount that I travel A LOT in the last ten years. And with more traveling comes a suitcase full of mistakes and a carry-on bag full of lessons. WHAT A CUTE SENTENCE.

Let's see if I can even remember all of my stupidity. I've left every possible charger in oh so many hotel rooms. I've gotten to the airport only to realize I'd left my wallet back at a friend's apartment. I've booked flights for the wrong days and only noticed once I got to the airline ticket counter. Most recently, I left my entire purse at the departure gate. MY ENTIRE PURSE. I only found out after I had boarded the plane and tried to find my credit card to pay for a drink. I've had to use body wash as my "shampoo," gum as my "toothpaste," and toilet seat covers as my "tampons" (that was a rough one, literally).

Traveling is amazing because you meet people, you see things, you open yourself up to life-changing experiences, BLAH BLAH BLAH. The other side of traveling is that there are so many uncontrollable factors that force you to problem-solve and adapt. I've learned that travel is a lot like changing a baby's diaper. When it goes well, it's wonderful and refreshing—when it doesn't, it's a sh*t storm. This probably isn't the best analogy. To be honest, I've never changed a baby's diaper. It's just that I respect babies too much to embarrass them like that. (Is it possible to donate your reproductive organs? I know I won't be needing mine.)

Here are some things I've learned over the years that might help you set yourself up for travel success.

1. **Pack deodorant.** You can tell I'm very, very serious about this. Like I've already said, deodorant can be perfume. If you've mismanaged your "get-ready time," deodorant is an instant shower!

2. **Always remember the underwear and socks.** If I had a nickel for every time I've had to endure dirty underwear or dirty socks while

away, I could probably buy a Subway sandwich right now. Six-inch. No, not the combo meal. I'm not THAT forgetful.

3. Assume your plane has no Wi-Fi. Remember to bring some source of batteryless/technologyless entertainment. MAYBE A BOOK????

4. Give yourself more time than you assume. I'm still struggling with this step. This is when being a fearful human is actually helpful. Always assume car tires will burst, gas tanks will run dry, or someone will oversleep. If those things don't happen and you get to your destination early, you get to reward yourself with something! You are both your own kindergarten teacher and well-behaved kindergarten student!

5. What's going on with your feet? Remember you have to take your shoes off at airport security in front of everyone else. This is another tip I keep learning the hard way. My feet are awful always (see: photo—I'm sorry). And when I have to fly I usually throw on any shoes that don't have laces so I don't have to be the Security Struggler. Socks are always an afterthought for me and I need to readjust that thought process. Again, I'm sorry.

6. Look up the weather in your destination city. When I see a guy wearing shorts in cold weather I don't assume he mispacked, I assume he's an "I've-got-something-to-prove" asshole. Maybe I'm awful. Either way, figure out the clothing situation.

7. Target has a really great travel section. Just saying.

8. You're not going to meet your fiancé on the plane, so you can look like a human gremlin. And if you do meet your fiancé, at least you'll know they love you for your base-level monster self. LOVE!

9. Dry shampoo, dry shampoo, dry shampoo. If you're a lady or man of long hair with a busy travel schedule, this is the most wonderful friend for you. It's like a padded bra for your hair. Allow it to present a false truth to your friends and strangers! Fun!

10. Always bring headphones. Even if you have nothing to plug them into, you can fake it so you don't have to listen to the strange woman next to you tell you about her concerns about her sister-in-law's recent weight gain.

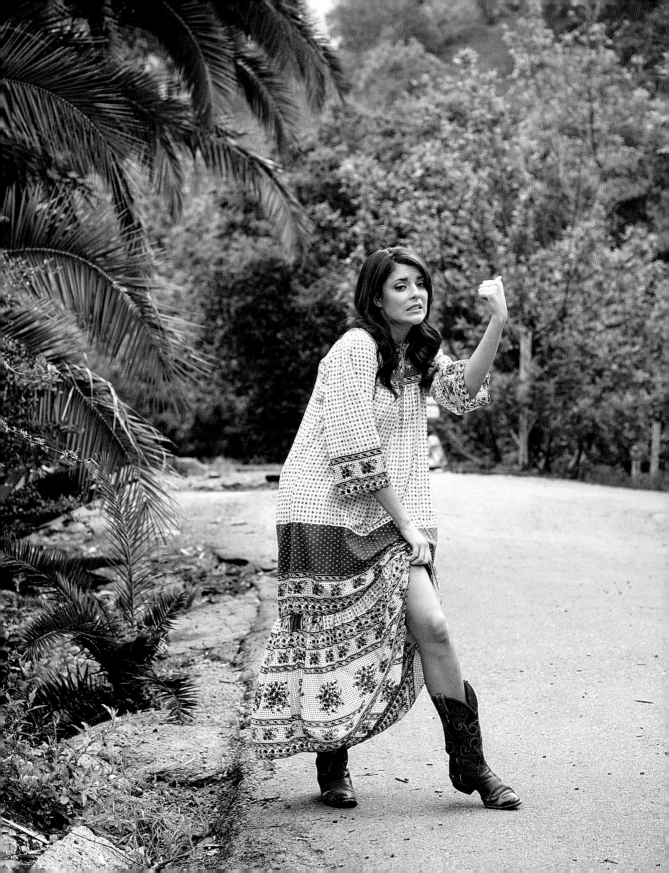

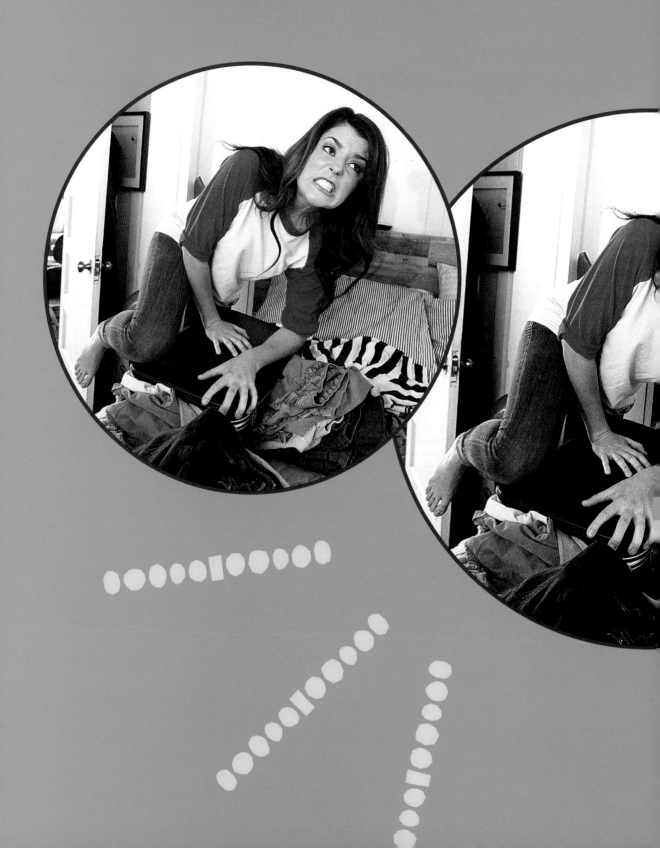

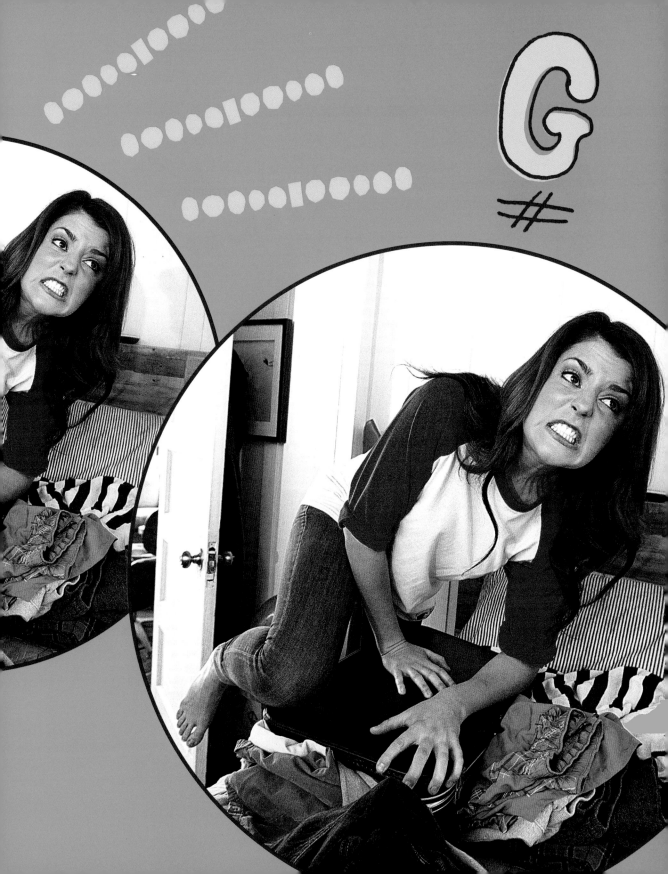

11. **SOCKS!** Wearing clean socks on an airplane is one of life's simple pleasures. I only know this because one time I saw the cutest British girl on a flight back from London and she was super dolled up in a dress and heels and looked like she stepped out of a Topshop ad and all I could think was, *Oh, you are NOT going to be comfortable on this ten-hour flight*. And, as if she could hear my inner monologue, she got up and walked to the bathroom with a bag and came back out in adorable sweatpants and an oversized shirt and the thickest, most comfortable-looking socks I'd ever seen. *OH SNAP. THIS GIRL KNOWS HOW TO TRAVEL*. And then she put on her neck pillow, turned on her computer already preset with movies and watched and fell asleep until right before we landed, and then she made her way back to the bathroom to change into the SUPER CUTE outfit she boarded the plane with. She was everything I could ever aspire to be.

12. **Precharge your electronics before you go.** And also make an attempt to preload them with movies and shows you want to watch.

Five things you should always travel with in your carry-on bag:

1. Money/plastic things that give you access to money
2. Chargers
3. A goddamn positive attitude
4. ID
5. Deodorant (you saw this coming)

Turns out airport Wi-Fi is always terrible and you won't be able to download them at your gate. I've missed out on so many really special episodes of *The Real Housewives* that way. What a waste. And don't forget your chargers! Double check.

13. **3.4 ounces is the max liquid you can pack in a carry-on!!!!** I think. Unless they changed it. They do that. Look up the number. I've been embarrassed so many times by TSA agents removing my spray-tan bottle and asking me if I knew that this was over the legal fluid ounce limit. Once they shamed me in front of a Texas family with real tans. And don't forget to take your water out of your bag before you get to security. Please don't be that person. You hate that person.

14. **Go through your bags BEFORE you get to security to make sure you took out that thing.** I don't know how much more I need to say here. You know your own secrets.

15. **You don't HAVE to check a bag.** And then you don't have to wait at baggage claim! I only recently figured this one out. I'm an idiot. Yes, all you fellow idiots out there, having to wait at baggage claim SUCKS. It feels like a very mild prank. You're thinking, *Did I misinterpret the baggage claim gate number? Was that person in the pleated khakis on my flight? Was that DOG on my flight? HOW DID I MISS THAT DOG ON THE FLIGHT?*

16. **Always sit near the front of a plane.** This is a tip I've only recently learned. You're close to bathrooms and the flight attendants, who can sneak you another drink/bag of chips. And you get off the plane first, which is the BEST.

17. MAKE FRIENDS WITH THE FLIGHT ATTENDANTS. I was recently on a flight with my friend Mamrie and my German friend Flula and our flight attendant (SHOUT-OUT TO MICHAEL ON JETBLUE!) was the greatest. He was flamboyant and hilarious and so wonderful. We made a few jokes with him as we boarded and when we officially introduced ourselves and ordered our drinks, he gave us two airplane bottles each along with our mixers. It's the little things. I hope you're reading this, Michael, you were great. (The best part of the story is that I went to the bathroom and on the way ordered a third round for each of us, but Mamrie wanted to switch up her order to a Corona and when I told Michael he was like, "OOOOH, MOONFACE WANTS A CORONA?" and I was like, "Moonface?" and he was like, "YEAH, MOONFACE WANTS A CORONA?" And I nodded and peed (in the bathroom) and went back to my seat and realized Mamrie was wearing a phases-of-the-moon sweatshirt. Ohhhh, moon PHASE wants a Corona. God, he was great.

18. Those neck pillow things look stupid but seriously work.

19. The in-flight security safety cards always have the most ridiculous graphics. Treat yourself to a giggle. Truly. Take a look.

20. Don't lean your chair back. You really don't need to. By nature airplanes are the most uncomfortable—leaning a chair back isn't going to make you content, it's going to make you an asshole. If you really NEED to get those ten to twenty extra reclining degrees, at least buy the person behind you a drink.

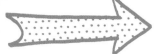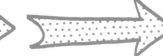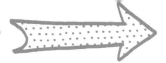

21. Don't be the person eating tuna on the plane. No explanation needed.

22. Wear your hoodie backward if you're sleeping in public, so no one has to see your gaping mouth and you don't have to breathe in everyone else's plane farts.

23. Water is a neat thing to consume while traveling. And just in general. Apparently it "keeps us alive."

24. SNACKS! Get them, have them, buy them. Snacks and traveling go together like my mouth and a basket of french fries.

25. Make up games! Whether you're in a plane, car, train, boat, or on a camel, stupid games are a great way to pass the time. F*ck-marry-kill: the Disney characters version is always a fun time.

26. If you're crossing the border you really don't have to create an elaborate story to explain to border control. You can tell them the truth. When my friends and I crossed the border from Canada into the U.S. during a small comedy tour, we got so nervous about how we'd explain why there were so many tuxedo onesies in our car and what we were planning on doing with the hamburger costume. We spent a couple hours trying to figure out if we'd say we were visiting friends, or that we were road tripping, or that one of our relatives' last dying wish was that we travel from Canada into the U.S. down the West Coast. By the time we got to the border the officer looked at our passports, completely disregarded our nervous,

goody-goody faces, and let us through. What a waste of a great relatives'-dying-wish story. Until next time, border control.

27. AAA gives hotel discounts! This is something I learned about last year and really want to let you know about! I had no idea! If you're on the road with no plan and you need to stay at the next hotel you see (been there—I've driven cross-country three times) and you have a AAA card, you can usually get 10 to 20 percent off the price if you ask about it. A hotel won't normally promote this. Your coupon-clipping mom/aunt will be so proud of you.

28. A hotel can be judged by its toiletries. If they're good, use them (or hide them!) and try to get housekeeping to replace them before you leave so you can take some for the road. And with that I will never be allowed in another hotel. Unless you have terrible toiletries! I'm looking at you, Motel 6.

29. Chain hotels are great! BUT figure out the chain no-bedbugs hotels. Assess chain hotels like you would assess a chain restaurant. Read reviews, listen to what the angriest Yelper has to say, and realize they're 60 percent over-exaggerating and take it from there. Sometimes you shouldn't order the tuna tartar at a restaurant in Oklahoma. If they have sheets you can sleep under without having to take a shower when you wake up, then COOL. Keep going.

30. You can squat in a hotel room longer than your original checkout time. I hate that I'm advocating this. From what I've heard, AND I DON'T KNOW FOR SURE, THIS IS A RUMOR (see: Lindsay Lohan's music video), you can stay in a hotel room longer than your checkout time if you (responsibly) ask for a later checkout time or (irresponsibly) linger in your room and tell them you have food poisoning from the hotel SHRIMP COCKTAIL. If you're sick from their food they have to keep you. Like an orphan!

31. Always go out the first night of your trip. Always. Even if you're so exhausted, just force yourself to have the tiniest amount of fun times. You never know when an emergency (anything from breaking a bone to your water breaking to a surprise new season of *Breaking Bad*) might happen and you'll have to leave before you had expected. Make sure you get your money's (or someone else's money's) worth.

32. Save chains for tires and prison fights. Try to find the one place in town that isn't a chain restaurant. It's usually delightfully representative of that area and offers something other than mozzarella sticks. And if they do offer the mozz sticks, they're probably better than T.G.I. Friday's. Oops.

33. Pack to leave the night before. My friends and I have developed a scientific travel system called "drunk packing." Basically, the night before we leave a place, we turn activities that usually aren't fun into FUN! If you pack when you're buzzed, it's a great time and you wake up with the work done. Your sober morning self only has to make sure you didn't miss anything. As I was writing this chapter, I realized that I had to call a hotel in London, because I left my wallet in the hotel room. Don't worry, I took everything out of it except my driver's license. SO DUMB. Please learn from my mistakes.

34. Find people you love to travel with and travel with them! #travel

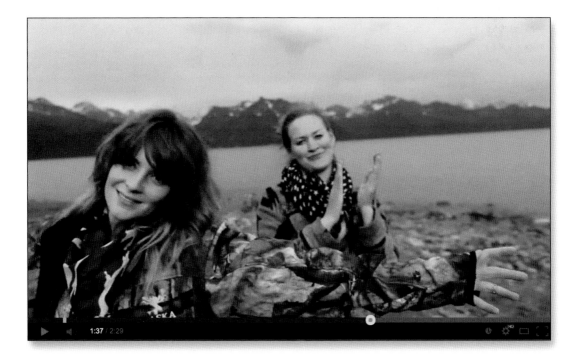

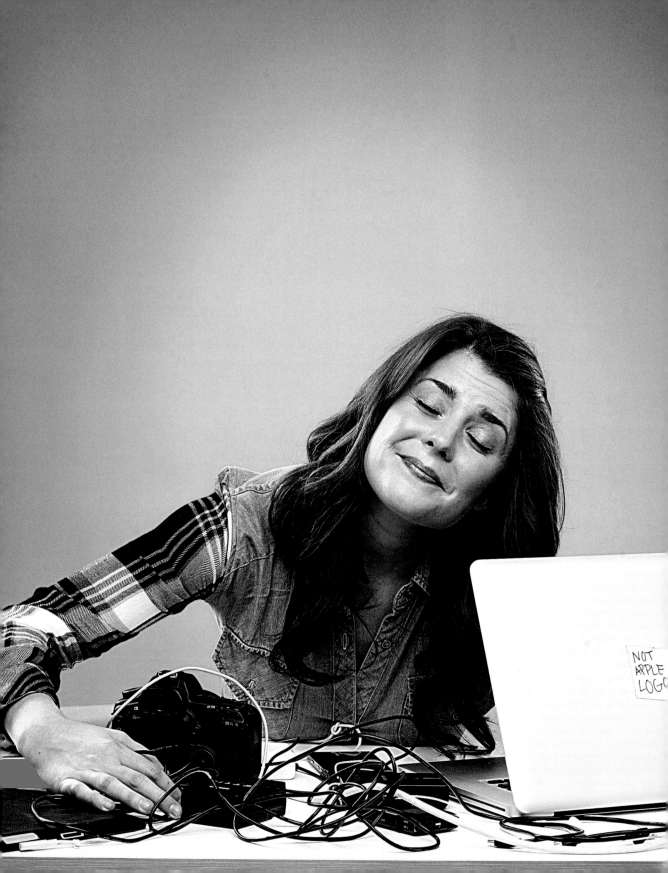

20 TIPS FOR LIVING ONLINE

I looked it up on the Internet—it's true, I'm a Millennial. The fact that I Googled the definition of "Millennial" proves I'm one of them.

When I was in seventh grade my family installed the Internet for the very first time on our only computer, a clunky desktop. It was a magical experience. We dialed up, it took *minutes*, and then my mom emailed my aunt via her brand-new Yahoo! email account. We immediately called her to make sure the email went through. And it did! What was this wizardry? I was ALL IN.

The Internet, turns out, is an introvert's paradise. I have two brothers, so we had to share time on the computer. Luckily, my younger brother was slightly too young and too into "books" at the time to appreciate the wonderfulness that was the World Wide Web, so the fight was always between my older brother, who only wanted to

play Diablo, and me, who only wanted to use AOL Instant Messenger and sign in to Yahoo! chat rooms to catfish people, before I even knew what catfishing was.

My middle school/high school after-school activities consisted of track and field and creating elaborate characters online to talk to people in chat rooms. I was a home-schooled boy from Wisconsin, a postgrad from Portland, a dental hygienist from Maine. Nothing got pervy, I just wanted to screw with people and see what they'd believe and what they'd want to talk about. Turns out 98 percent of people just wanted to cyber. Cool job, humanity.

When I graduated high school and went to college, MySpace and Facebook became part of my world—I was done for. I remember discovering MySpace for the first time via my roommate. After I created a profile and checked to see which of my friends were already on the site, I found out that my own boyfriend of a year already had a profile. Turns out he had been active on the site for months. He knew how much I loved the Internet; why didn't he fill me in?

"You've known about MySpace?" I asked.

"Yeah," he said.

"Why didn't you tell me about it?"

"I dunno."

He was a great conversationalist. That should have been a #redflag.

As I went through college, I got more and more into the Internet. My senior year I found a funny female vlogging duo named Beth and Val who became my inspiration/introduction to vlogging. They recorded themselves on their MacBook iSight camera answering a question submitted from their audience over email. They hilariously answered the question over the course of two minutes using *jump cuts*. This changed my entire world.

A jump cut is an editing term for an abrupt transition from one scene to another. Jump cuts make jokes funnier, make mundane conversations more interesting, and overall make dull people seem like they have personality. I was ALL IN.

Immediately after discovering Beth and Val, I made my roommate vlog with me. And now, eight years later, I make my living online, recording my face quacking at a camera. I spend an average of probably six to ten hours online every day via my computer or phone. That sounds awful. But it's my job. And also my hobby. I LOVE THE INTERNET. Even when I try to take a break, all I want to do is check my Instagram feed. I'm sure a lot of psychologists might say that this is unhealthy behavior. To that I say, SIKE-ologists! I'm participating in a community! I liked five pictures of French bulldogs on Instagram this morning, what have you done today?

Because I've spent the past few years living and breathing online, I've discovered a few tips to help those who were born with or without Wi-Fi.

1. **Privacy: keep some of your personal life offline.** Find a balance between the Internet and IRL. It'll keep you sane. Or closer to it.

2. **Friends CAN be made via the WWW.** Just proceed with caution. I have little room to speak on this; my first real romantic relationship was maintained via AOL Instant Messenger. But I met him in the human world first. So I knew I wasn't being social-media-swindled. I've had a lot of fans meet up for the first time at some of my live shows and it's always a wonderful thing to hear about/see in my Tumblr tags. Like!

3. Don't drink and digital. There has to be an app that shuts you off after you make a certain number of spelling mistakes in a tweet before sending it.

4. An email signature tricks people into thinking you're a professional.

5. You can learn a lot about a person based on their mobile email signature. Mine used to say, "Sent from my eyefone (sp?)." SO CLEVER! HIRE ME.

6. Keep your personal confrontations off the Internet. We get it; you're opinionated about stuff. We get it; you want attention for it. We get it; the Internet is a public forum from which you can collect that attention. But, like, why? Try to enjoy something in your life.

7. Subtweeting is for tweens. This is related to the last tip. According to Urban Dictionary (my source for most "youth talk"), a subtweet is: "A tweet (message posted on the website Twitter) that mentions a Twitter member without using their actual username. Usually employed for negative or insulting tweets." So dumb. Either talk to that person about your feelings or get a LiveJournal (I'm old).

8. Manage your time. The Internet is a time vacuum. It will suck all of your time away from you. Try to stay aware of how much you're giving up. Look up from time to time.

9. Manage your brand. This tip isn't just specific to those who wish to pursue some sort of online content creator profession. Take time to fully understand what you have to offer the Internet. What's your point of view? Who's your audience? How can you speak to them authentically and genuinely? I could talk for hours on this subject. I've limited myself to these few sentences. If you'd like me to develop some sort of longer-form workshop, just say the word and I'll add it to my three-page to-do list.

10. Be careful about what you "like." People can see that stuff. If you like that girl's TwitPic of her thong or all those girls' butt photos on Instagram, I can see that. And I will judge you. I'm sorry.

11. Beware of people who voluntarily post bikini/shirtless photos. This is general life advice. They have something to prove.

12. **Yes, those black-and-white photos of your wedding and/or child are very beautiful.** Do you feel validated? Okay, now stop.

13. **You will get judged by your Instagram filter.** X-Pro II? Really? Step up your game. You're better than that.

14. **If you have numbers in your profile name/handle, you won't be taken seriously.** I'm sorry, that's just life. And generally speaking, it's a lot harder for people to remember your contact info. Unless the numbers are 6 and 9 together—then I give you two thumbs up (the butt).

15. **Google it, don't tweet it.** If you have a question about something, just look it up. If you want popular opinion, tweet it. Sorry to sound annoyed, but I don't want to have to figure out what you're allergic to based on a gross selfie you posted on Twitter.

16. **Follow ALL the dogs on Instagram.** This is pretty much a tip applicable for every part of your life. They are the best and I spend a good portion of my "workday" looking through dog Instagram photos. One day, I was waiting for my video to upload, and while waiting I checked Instagram on my phone and started following two new dog accounts. People saw this (see: tip #10) and thought I wasn't posting my video yet, because I was too busy looking at pictures of dogs. They were half right. I regret nothing.

17. **Work in offline mode.** My friend Hannah found an app that allows her to download her in-box so when she knows she won't be connected to Wi-Fi she can work offline and respond to unanswered emails. She can compose full email responses and set them to send and as soon as she gets reconnected to Wi-Fi *they all send*. It's one of the more brilliant things I've seen her do. And I've seen her steal a stool from a bar and carry it to her apartment half a mile away.

18. **Make your passwords the dumbest.** And change them every few months. This is common knowledge, but hacking is getting scary (you can't spell "scary" without "cray"). Keep a private list somewhere of all your passwords, because you'll forget. Sorry I'm not giving you enough credit. You're wonderful.

19. **Don't let negative comments get to you.** When I first started making Web videos, I would read every comment and take it to heart. HI, DEPRESSION. Eventually I started picturing every negative commenter living an unfulfilling life and instead of feeling bad about myself, I felt sad for them. Because that's pretty much the truth. People only make other people feel bad when they feel bad about themselves. It's in the Bible somewhere, I think.

20. **Don't send pictures of your privates to anyone online.** Ever. Done. Period. It's why they're called "privates."

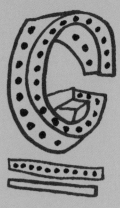

You've made it through the book! Unless you're looking at the last page before actually reading any of it because you don't allow yourself to properly experience a good thing. It's okay; there are other books you could read to help with that.

I hope this book made you smile at least once. I hope maybe you learned something you didn't know before. I hope it brought some form of happiness to your day that you didn't expect or that you desperately needed. If it didn't do any of that stuff . . . well . . . uh . . . maybe go read *The Fault in Our Stars* again?

eeeee

collar tug

You rule it. Thanks for doing life with me!

THANK YOU TO...

...MY EDITOR, LAUREN, WHO'S BEEN UNBELIEVABLY PATIENT AND ENCOURAGING AND HAS ALLOWED ME TO USE THE WORD "DIARRHEA" FOUR TIMES IN PRINT.

...MY PHOTOGRAPHER, ROBIN, WHO'S STUPIDLY TALENTED (DUH!) AND DIDN'T THINK TWICE WHEN I TOLD HER I NEEDED A LOAF OF BREAD SO SHE COULD PHOTOGRAPH ME HITTING SOMEONE IN THE FACE WITH IT.

...MY BROTHER, TIM, FOR CONTRIBUTING THE FOREWORD TO THE BOOK AND FOR ALWAYS MAKING ME UGLY-FACE-SCREAM-LAUGH UNTIL I CRY.

...MY BEST FRIENDS, HANNAH AND MAMRIE, FOR HANDLING MY CRAZY WHILE I WROTE THE BOOK IN A LIMITED AMOUNT OF TIME, AND FOR ALWAYS INSPIRING ME TO CHASE A BETTER, DUMBER (IN THE BEST WAY) VERSION OF MYSELF.

...MY MOM, FOR SPRINKLING HER PERSONAL WORDS OF WISDOM THROUGHOUT THE BOOK, FOR GETTING OVERLY EXCITED ABOUT EVEN MY SMALLEST SUCCESSES, AND FOR BEING AVAILABLE WHENEVER I NEED HER TO CHEER ME UP, KEEP ME GROUNDED, OR FIND UNFLATTERING CHILDHOOD PHOTOS.

...MY DAD, STEPMOM, AND STEPDAD, FOR THE CONSTANT SUPPORT, LOVE, AND OFFERS TO HELP ME MOVE.

...MY "YOU," FOR BEING 100 PERCENT.

...MY AUDIENCE, FOR F*CKING RULING IT.

...MY DOG, GOOSE, FOR BEING AN ADORABLE WHIRLING DERVISH OF LOVE AND HILARITY. IT'D BE COOL IF YOU COULD READ THIS.

...MY PROFESSIONAL TEAM—ESPECIALLY MY MANAGER, KEN, AND MY AGENT, ERIN—FOR PUSHING ME FORWARD AND APPROVING OF MY INSANITY.

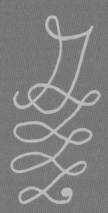

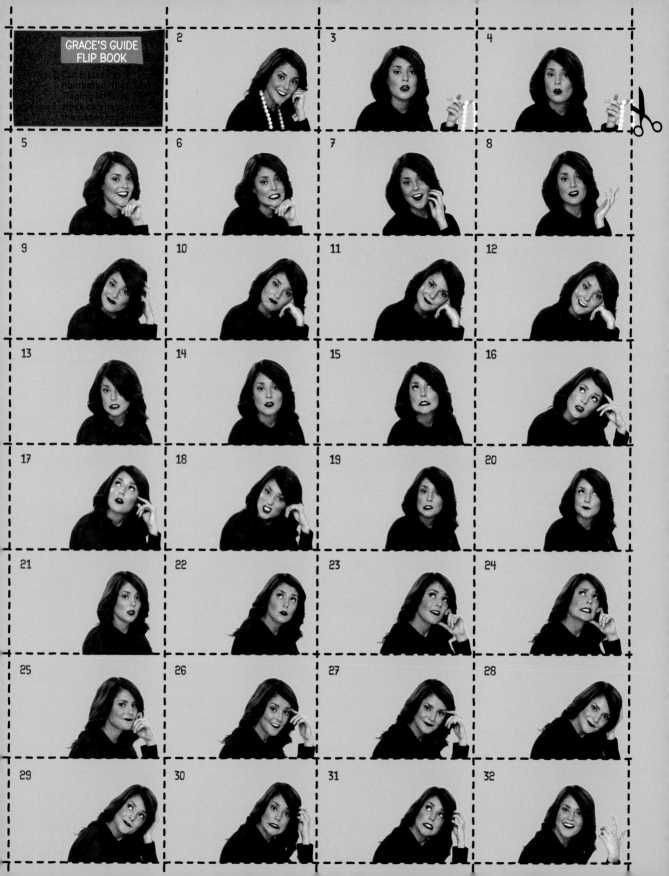

GRACE'S GUIDE
FLIP BOOK

Cut & stack in numbered, then flip. Taping the inside of the stack can help keep the pages together.

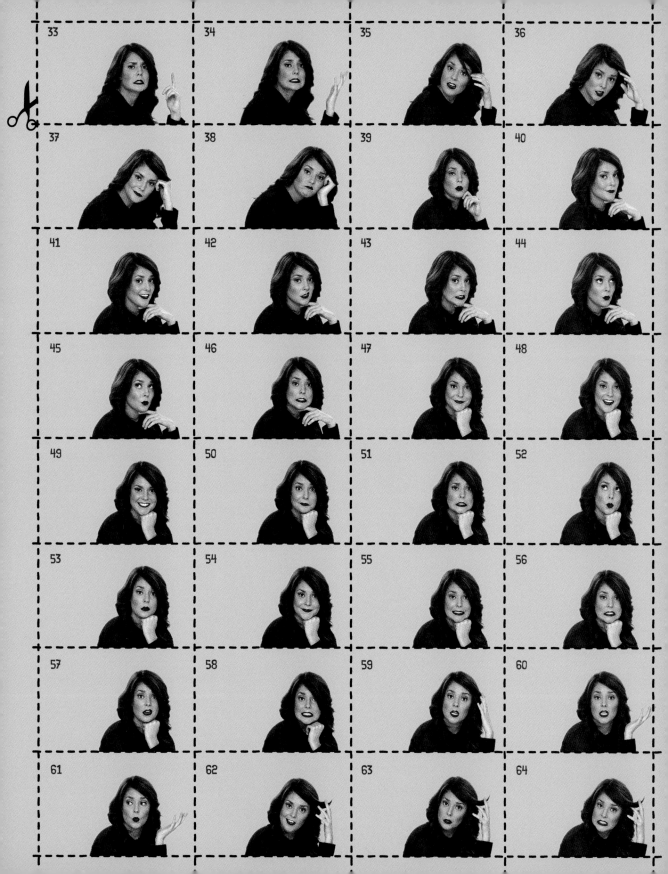

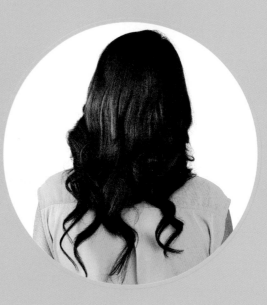

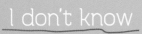
I don't know